Health
Mindset
and
Lifespan

Health Mindset *and* Lifespan

LONGEVITY NEW SCIENCE SUPERPOWERS FOR HEALTHY LIVES.

Living younger with a long healthspan and a longevity diet; the power to reduce stress and detox your mindset; and the new science in lifespan technology.

HOWARD E. WELLER

First Edition

Published by Key Focus Publishers Ltd

Key Focus Publishers has the right to use the author's name
Howard E. Weller
www.howardeweller.com

DISCLAIMER

Although the author and publisher have made every effort to ensure that the information in this book was correct at press time, the author and publisher do not assume and hereby disclaim any liability to any party for any loss, damage, disruption, or illness caused by errors or omissions, whether such errors or omissions result from negligence, accident, or any other cause.

The publisher and the author are providing this book and its contents on an "as is" basis and make no representations or warranties of any kind with respect to this book or its contents. The publisher and the author disclaim all such representations and warranties, including but not limited to warranties of healthcare for a particular purpose. In addition, the publisher and the author assume no responsibility for errors, inaccuracies, omissions, or any other inconsistencies herein.

The content of this book is for informational purposes only and is not intended to diagnose, treat, cure, or prevent any condition or disease. You understand that this book is not intended as a substitute for consultation with a licensed practitioner. Please consult with your own physician or healthcare specialist regarding the suggestions and recommendations made in this book. The use of this book implies your acceptance of this disclaimer.

The publisher and the author make no guarantees concerning the level of success you may experience by following the advice and strategies contained in this book, and you accept the risk that results will differ for each individual. The testimonials and examples provided in this book show exceptional results, which may not apply to the average reader, and are not intended to represent or guarantee that you will achieve the same or similar results.

CONTENTS

INTRODUCTION:

ARE YOU READY TO ADJUST TO THE NEW AGE?

Have you ever thought, "I don't have enough time!" What if you had longer to achieve your goals?

If you've picked up this book, the chances are you are a lover of life and want to live out your dreams. You are the kind of person who wants to make the most of the time you have. Days and weeks may roll by without too much fanfare, but I would imagine that you want to make the most of each year or plan for the coming years.

Ill-health may not normally be at the top of your worries, but this is often the most impactful. A set-back due to ill-health would be frustrating at the least, and life-threatening at the worst. If at all possible, you'll want to extend and look forward to the healthy years you have and do everything in your power to avoid long-term or age-related diseases.

It is possible you are feeling the effects of ageing in your body, and you are likely trying to treat yourself better, in order to slow down some of those effects. You may feel uneasy about the rise in social media use, and the way it makes you and others feel about the effects of ageing. And you've probably researched a little already into healthcare options that are thought to keep us young.

I'm here to tell you, first and foremost, you're not alone; and secondly, the ability to feel younger and live longer is entirely within your grasp.

I've always been interested in what we can do in our lifetime. From a young age, I thought I had a window of around thirty years or so before retiring, but that wasn't a satisfying vision. I want to keep going for longer, to live more with my life. Even when I was a teenager, I would seek out news articles, TV programmes and expert opinions that indicated there was more to life expectancy than meets the eye, giving me a longer window for a healthy, productive lifespan. I've been drawn to thought leaders and visionaries that aim for moon shots, and people who design technologies that can improve the lives many. And most of all, I love doing the research, going through the academic papers, exploring where the scientists believe there is potential for further study. I like to determine where the scientists have been holding back their optimism.

As a student, I excelled at mathematics – using a set of equations that could describe or dictate how the world around us works. I studied this in so much detail that I achieved such high exam results in my Master of Mathematics degree that I was top of my year at one of the leading university mathematics departments in the UK. My particular focus was on applied mathematics, looking at the natural laws behind quantum theory, fluid dynamics, and biological mathematics. This led to a fascinating study of the natural world, culminating in a dissertation in mathematical neuroscience that reviewed the models of how neurons in the brain interact with each other and achieve synchronicity. I was only 21 turning 22, and already exposed to the burgeoning field of biological science.

After graduating, I started to work in the City of London as a corporate finance analyst at Close Brothers. This led to a position as an analyst in investment management at Frank Investments. However, after finding the urge to be re-immersed in the rich academic world again, I applied to the University of Cambridge, where I was lucky enough to be awarded a scholarship to study for an MBA at the Judge Business School. This was a truly enjoyable course. While at Cambridge, I decided to specialise in Social Innovation, which looked at the broader context of business, leadership and values. This curriculum led me to explore more relevant organisations for nature, social good and the planet. This is an area I continue to explore and is very relevant with the increasing focus and accountability of companies and their environmental and social impacts.

Whatever I work on, I dive into the detail, and research as much as I can to understand and distil the information; it comes from an inherent interest in people, in science, and in nature.

With regard to longevity, one of the early signs for me that more was possible was a TV program featuring a 55-year-old man with the physiology of a 20-year-old. He and his wife were on a calorie restrictive diet which seemed to be helping their bodies maintain astounding youth. Delving into the sector with more enthusiasm, I was able to start unearthing how our cells have inbuilt systems to repair. These systems are often triggered by times of hardship. My interest and knowledge bloomed from there onward.

This book is a summary of some of my findings, captured in a format that I hope is easy to understand and enjoy. The contents are a decade's worth of interest and research into a sector that has dramatically changed to be unrecognisable from when I was a child. There are astounding advances in our understanding of the body and mind, which I believe is relevant to you regardless of whether you are young or "old".

There are some estimates that the *average* lifespan in ancient Greek and Roman times was as little as 20-35 years. These figures are skewed though by the incredibly high rates of infant mortality. Historians believe that from around 1500-1800, life expectancy in Europe was roughly 30-40 years of age.[1]

Life expectancy has more than doubled since 1900. This is due to the elimination of diseases such as typhoid, smallpox, and scarlet fever. There have also been massive improvements in hygiene and sanitation.

---

[1] Basaraba, S. (2020, April 24). *How Has Longevity Changed Throughout History?* Verywell Health.

There is some variability among comparable countries, though.[2] And there are significant inequalities in life expectancy across the globe. These inequalities also exist within countries according to income level unfortunately. Continuous scientific breakthroughs in medicine will help bring better health to people with lower income, and philanthropic missions are key to support these areas in the meantime.

In recent years, many ground-breaking studies demonstrate that current mainstream ideas about lifespan are out-of-date. Lifespan figures we grew up with, which have barely changed in decades are based purely on historical cases and don't consider the developments in science and medicine, our own personal learning, and our daily lifestyle habits.

I would go as far as to say that our current mindset about ageing is preventing us from outliving the statistics. This is because we may have heard of such improvements available to us but haven't updated our longer-term view. Without reassessing the long lifespan that we are hoping and likely to achieve, we are holding back our health, holding back our ambitions, holding back our enjoyment of time with family and friends.

If, so far, this is hard to believe, then please humour me for one moment. Imagine, if you will, the possibility that in thirty years' time you'll still have as much physical ability, energy and youthfulness as you do now. Close your eyes, take a long breath and focus on only that. Your health will be as good as it is now for another thirty years. Notice the physiological reactions within your body, within your mind. Do you feel lighter? Did your shoulders relax? Did your mind slow down? Did you feel a sense of relief or elation? Did you feel calm?

It is possible you didn't feel any of these things, but I suspect that if you have an interest in this topic by picking up this book, the idea of living a little bit longer than commonly reported figures suggest, has invoked a sense of *something* pleasant within you.

---

[2] Kamal, R. (2019, December 23). *Health System Tracker*. Health System Tracker.

A lot of our stress comes from the feeling of not having enough time. In fact, there's even a name for it: time anxiety.[3] We can experience time anxiety on a number of different levels. It can manifest in a fear of being late to everyday appointments and activities, or it can contribute to a negative, defeatist attitude, or it can trigger existential dread. If we allow ourselves to focus on the bigger picture, the grand scheme of our life's opportunity, we can put those things that trigger our time anxiety into a new, hopefully more freeing, perspective.

Becoming less anxious in our day-to-day life is a giant step towards making that increased longevity a greater possibility. And bear in mind, this is a fact we have only truly realised in the last couple of decades. There are many other recent advancements in our understanding that can contribute to our longevity. In this book, we will discuss the key developments that you can take advantage of now, to extend your own lifespan.

The ultimate goal of this book is to shift your mindset. If you can shift your mindset, you'll be able to adopt a healthier lifestyle and be ready to spot future advances that reinforce the learnings from this book. More recent scientific study tells us we can greatly improve the quality of our life at all ages, especially from our mid-life onwards. But our current mindset probably doesn't factor this in. This historic mindset will hold back our life expectancy from fulfilling its true potential.

Throughout this book, we will discuss the latest developments in science and technology, as well as our accompanying levels of understanding. It is my goal that, by the time you reach the end, your mindset will have adapted to the very real idea that you have many more quality years of life ahead of you than you think. And that higher quality years will be realised not only in the long term but in the short term too. You will be released from restrictive and limiting beliefs about ageing, and this will hopefully open up opportunities you might have previously dismissed.

---

[3] Raypole, C. (2020, August 31). *Time Anxiety*. Healthline.

With an up-to-date mindset in relation to our lifespan, we can subtly (or dramatically) shift the way we feel day-to-day and take instant steps to make that greater longevity a reality.

The key areas we need to focus on in order to revise our beliefs about lifespan and longevity are the healthcare solutions that are available now; our mental wellbeing; diets that reduce inflammation and environmental impact on our bodies; and scientific breakthroughs that completely change our understanding about ageing.

All I need you to do now, at the outset of reading this book, is to open your mind and accept that it is possible to change our mindset and benefit from the physiological benefits this can bring.

According to Elissa Epel, a University of California professor who studies stress and ageing, it simply "comes down to daily behaviour and the choices we make. We have a growing set of studies of people from around the world showing that ageing is not just an aspect of genetics but of how we live." All we have to do is make a decision to take steps to adopt a lifestyle that is more conducive to longevity[4].

The longer you hold on to rigid beliefs that you are only going to live to your early eighties at the most, the more opportunities you could be missing. Missing opportunities to create a life you love now and will continue to love well into older age. Not only that, if you hold onto beliefs that could be – directly, or indirectly – causing you mental stress, you're not helping your body to ready itself for a longer lifespan.

By the time you reach the end of this book, you will know the key elements that will help you to prolong your life, and how to leverage them to your advantage. You will have a clearer understanding of how scientific advancements have made it possible for us to better manage the effects of ageing, whether they are within our reach or not quite yet. And it is my aim that you will feel confident of your longevity, with a mindset that has been reprogrammed to support this.

---

[4] Kluger, J. (2015, February 12). *How your Mindset Can Change How You Age*. Time.

In short, if you read the following chapters with an open mind and a willingness to allow your perspective on ageing to shift, then this book will change your life.

CHAPTER 1:
UPFRONT POWER OF MINDSET

Our mindset is incredibly powerful when it comes to our outlook and decisions. I want to address this right away as it will likely be key to further progress toward a more fulfilled life. Consider this chapter a warm up exercise to get you ready for the detail of longevity.

How does mindset work?

Whenever we learn something new, our brain creates a 'neural pathway', a quick route to the new information that becomes more and more deeply ingrained the more frequently we use the pathway. For example, when we learn to brush our teeth for the first time, the brain creates a neural pathway. Each time we brush our teeth, the pathway becomes stronger and more imprinted on our minds. Pretty soon, we can brush our teeth with our eyes closed, or without hardly thinking about it. This is the way we form habits, by doing one thing – or a series of things – repeatedly, until we can do it without even thinking about it.

Luckily, our brains also possess neuroplasticity, which means we have the ability to change these pathways if we want to. It can take a lot of work, especially if certain habits, thoughts or opinions have become deeply imprinted on our minds. For example, if every day for twenty years you have told yourself that you don't like the shape of your nose, you can give yourself a different message multiple times each day, but it may take some time – weeks, months even – for your brain to rewrite that neural pathway. But with desire, determination and a regular practice, it is possible, and that's the most important point to take away from this.

The thing that comes before the determination to change the neural pathways, however, is the attitude. If you don't set out with a determined attitude and intention, it will be hard for you to influence your neural pathways.

Our mindset has incredible power over the way we live, the way we behave, how we find happiness, and how we heal and flourish. Even if we want to behave a certain way or think a certain way, a negative mindset can override these intentions. Having a particular, more positive, mindset, can lead to success. In this instance, success is willing to learn about longevity, so that you may be able to have a longer and healthier life[5].

Having a 'growth' or a 'learning' mindset throughout the course of your life can prove to be the difference between succeeding in life and achieving the goals you set for yourself, or not – to be frank, the likelihood is that life will be rather limited. According to an article by Carol Dweck for the Harvard Business Review, "Individuals who believe their talents can be developed (through hard work, good strategies, and input from others) have a growth mindset. They tend to achieve more than those with a more fixed mindset (those who believe their talents are innate gifts). This is because they worry less about looking smart and they put more energy into learning."[6]

Anyone can benefit from a greater understanding of how our mindsets work, and how we can use mindset to our advantage – successful business leaders included. The Brandon Hall Group, a human capital research and analyst firm conducted its research into leadership mindset by surveying 329 organisations. They identified four distinct types of mindset which were found to "affect leaders' ability to engage with others, navigate changes more successfully, and perform in their leadership roles more effectively"[7].

[5] Dweck, C. (2017b). Mindset - Updated Edition: Changing The Way You think To Fulfil Your Potential
[6] Dweck, C. (2016, January 13). *What Having a "Growth Mindset" Actually Means*. Harvard Business Review
[7] Gottfredson, R., & Reina, C. (2020, January 17). *To Be a Great Leader, You Need the Right Mindset*. Harvard Business Review

In their findings, success comes in the form of a mindset that is focussed on Growth, Learning, Deliberative, and Promotion.

Growth vs Fixed Mindsets: Having a growth mindset is to believe that people can change and grow their talent, skills and abilities. A fixed mindset comes from the belief that people can't. It is commonly thought that those with a growth mindset are more adaptable, resilient and able to weather challenges and setbacks better than others.

Learning vs Performance Mindsets. Someone with a learning mindset is thought to be motivated to develop their knowledge and skills. A performance mindset is more concerned with gaining positive feedback about achievements. This may seem counterintuitive, but the findings saw that leaders who can see the world as a learning opportunity, had a whole host of benefits in tackling business situations. These include a willingness to learn at a much deeper level, to seek out and incorporate feedback (or feedforward as we called it in Cambridge), exert more effort, have persistence, are more adaptable, are more willing to cooperate, and perform at a higher level.

Deliberative vs Implemental Mindsets. A deliberative mindset is associated with a greater receptiveness to all kinds of information to support actions and decision-making. An implemental mindset is where a person simply focuses on how to carry out a decision, thereby blinkering someone from additional information and ideas. Better decisions are made by deliberative mindset people because they are more accurate and less biased in the processing and decision making.

Promotion vs Prevention Mindsets. A promotion mindset is concerned with the pursuit of goals, gains and wins. A prevention mindset, on the other hand, focuses on avoiding loss at all costs. The former is more inclined towards positive thinking and are more open to change, the latter, negative with lower task performance and less persistence.

What these definitions tell us is that there are multiple types of mindset – positive and negative – which can help and hinder us in our progress through life. It's important to identify – if only loosely – your mindset type because then you can set about re-programming it, if need be, to be more open and receptive to new facts about lifespan and longevity. This can be easier than you think. I have some suggestions for you later in this chapter to help.

My understanding of those mindsets and from further reading around this subject, an ability to think that you can change and learn will help boost your positiveness throughout your life. Taking in as much information and considering why things are the way they are, will help you find more energy and persistence in the tasks that you set yourself. Even if it seems natural to limit the downside, it will be better if we can remain open to change, to allow ourselves to focus on the positive where at all possible.

In a study into the benefits of positive thinking, it was found that men and women with a more optimistic mindset benefitted from greater odds of living 14.9% longer or to 85 years old, respectively[8]. We'll look at this in more detail later in chapter 10.

Another study, which looked at optimism in relation to healthy ageing in women, found that optimistic women had a 23% greater likelihood of healthy ageing. According to the research, which analysed data from a study involving 33,326 women, "Higher optimism was associated with increased likelihood of healthy ageing, suggesting that optimism, a potentially modifiable health asset, merits further research for its potential to improve health in ageing."[9]

A further, large-scale study of 70,000 women and 1,400 men, featured in the *Proceedings of the National Academy of Sciences*, also links optimism with longer life. It concluded that, "For both men and women, higher levels of optimism were associated with a longer life

---

[8] Lee, L. O. (2019, September 10). *Optimism is associated with exceptional longevity in 2 epidemiologic cohorts of men and women.* PubMed.
[9] James, P. (2018, July 3). *Optimism and Healthy Ageing in Women.* PubMed.

span and "exceptional longevity," which the researchers defined as surviving to 85."

When it comes to mindset, I want to highlight some supporting foundations. We will cover longevity tips in plenty of detail later. But for now, here are some hopefully helpful suggestions that will boost your life.

I speak from experience when I say that cultivating a positive mindset is not only possible, but it can also be reasonably easy. I've listed below five tips that can help you move towards creating a more positive mindset. But, a word of advice, if you are entering into this completely new, just take things one step at a time (and with an open mind). You don't need to follow all these five tips every day – don't put that kind of pressure on yourself. Perhaps start by focusing on one of the tips each day for a week, and once you've created the early stages of a habit, try incorporating a second tip. Moving through these gradually might mean you stick with them longer.

Start the day with a positive affirmation

If you've never done this before, it might feel a little uncomfortable to repeat certain words to yourself at any opportune moment. So, choose something simple to begin with, such as 'I always look for the good in each day'. Repeat this affirmation to yourself whenever you remember to. Perhaps include this in your meditation practice if you do that regularly. You could always write it down on post-it notes and stick them around the house, the car or your desk, to remind yourself. It may take some practice but try to feel and believe those words as you repeat them. Over time, you'll start to notice that you are naturally seeking out the good in each day. Then you can move on to create other, clearer or more personal, affirmations.

Practice gratitude

Willie Nelson famously said, "When I started counting my blessings, my whole life turned around." There's a reason why many successful people cite gratitude as a key factor in their success. It is much easier to strive for something you want when you appreciate what you already have. Practising gratitude takes hardly any time at all. If you can remind yourself throughout the day to recognise something you are grateful for – someone giving up their spot in a queue for you, someone holding a door open for you, a nice compliment, a quick commute to work – then acknowledging that gratitude takes hardly any effort. But many find it easier to journal at the start or the end of each day, listing the things that have brought them happiness, even if fleeting. Try different ways of practising gratitude to see what works best for you.

Try to move your body every day

Just stretching each morning can make you feel better, by allowing oxygen to flow through your blood and tissues. Over time, you will also feel more flexible and less stiff and 'old'. If you can get outdoors every day, for a walk or run, or to play a sport, you will feel instantly fresher. The benefits of taking time to be outside in the fresh air, or in nature, are well-documented. The important thing to take away here is, you should try to make it a habit of it if you can. A little exercise or fresh air every day can have a substantial effect over the long term.

Exercise not only benefits the body, but it can also benefit the mind. According to Harvard Medical School, "The mental benefits of aerobic exercise have a neurochemical basis. Exercise reduces levels of the body's stress hormones, such as adrenaline and cortisol. It also stimulates the production of endorphins, chemicals in the brain that are the body's natural painkillers and mood elevators."

Also, breathing through your nose is really important as it will increase the flow of oxygen throughout the body. Taking large gasping breaths through your mouth actually has the opposite effect. So always try to keep that mouth shut and breathe easily through your nose, even if that means slowing down or exercising less vigorously.

Nourish yourself

Feed your body nutritious food and plenty of water. You need certain things to survive, even before you can thrive. All too often, we can jump to a quick-fix, fad diet that promises us greater energy or a more streamlined physique, but then neglect to give ourselves light, air and water. Our bodies can't function optimally, or fuel that all-important mindset unless those basic requirements are met.

Be mindful of self-talk and negative thoughts

Make a point each day of being conscious of your thoughts. Notice when you say something mean to yourself, or about another person or situation. Consciously reframe that thought in your mind and notice any changes in your body as you release that negativity. Becoming mindful of self-talk is one of the hardest things to do if you are not used to doing it. So, give yourself time to make a habit of noticing when you are leaning towards a negative thought, and be forgiving of yourself when you spot one that needs to be reframed. Old habits do die hard, and well-established neural pathways can take time to cover over while new paths are reinforced. Go easy on yourself as you adopt this practice.

The key to nurturing a positive mindset is to 'practice' until it becomes a habit. As Aristotle famously said: "We are what we repeatedly do." If you can begin to cultivate a more positive mindset, you are already streets ahead in terms of readiness to process some of the findings I'm about to put in front of you. That's all you really need to start adapting your mindset to the idea you can have a lot longer to live than you might think.

CHAPTER 2:
YOUR PURPOSE WILL TAKE YOU FAR

Those who know the purpose of their life, the things they want to achieve, where they want to go and how they can get there, tend to live a more meaningful existence than those who don't.[10]

It is often said that the benefits of having clear goals and direction for where we want our lives to go, help us to stay focused on the things that matter (and the things we enjoy), it makes us feel passionate about our dreams and achievements, it gives our lives clarity, helping us stay focused on important steps, it makes us feel gratified being able to see the results of our focus, and it makes us feel able to live a more value-based life.

You probably have some kind of goal outlined in your mind for the future. This could be a desire to be happy, and to have that happiness at a specific point in time or age. Or your goal might be to have lots of adventures and live a full life, or something you may have to save money for or wait until the kids have left home and you have greater freedom. Or you may have a goal to help and support people close to you, providing opportunities for them. All of these goals are wonderful and really important, in order to give you something to focus on and work towards.

Many of us know exactly what we're going to be doing for the rest of the day, the coming weekend, the next few months. In fact, many of

---

[10] Erin, S. (2019, September 20). *Your "Why" Matters: The 10 Benefits of Knowing Your Purpose in Life*. Goalcast.

us have heavily thumbed calendars and to-do lists of items we tick off every day. But not all of us take the time to think about what it is we want out of life – big picture. There's nothing inherently wrong with this, but the chances are, if you don't have some sort of vision (even one that changes and adapts as you grow and age) you may wake up in ten years' time and wonder what you've achieved or find that you've drifted into someone else's idea of what your life should be like. If you are unsure what your specific goals are, you are not alone.

The vision you create, or the specific goals you outline, do not need to be far-fetched or grand. They can be as small as making a point of appreciating your partner every day or trying out a new form of exercise each month. The important thing is taking the time to figure out who you are and what you want – it's amazing how many people really don't know this – and then plan to achieve things that fulfil you, in the short or long term.

Goals come in many forms. They can be focused on your professional life or personal life, your health and fitness, your sporting endeavours, your finances, your ongoing learning and education, your spiritual and philanthropic interests. While the goals don't have to border on unattainable, it is good to put a little ambition behind them, if only to re-tread the neural pathway that leads to your conviction that there are possibilities everywhere.[11]

There's a brilliant example of potentially the grandest of goals and what it meant to the people that set their sights upon it. Two of the United States founding fathers, John Adams and Thomas Jefferson, were instrumental in the forming of the United States Declaration of Independence in 1776. Their desire was to see the impacts of this creation of a new nation, and this gave purpose for their lives thereafter. On the 50th anniversary of the Declaration of Independence, they both died within a few hours of each other. At the time of their deaths on July 4, 1826, their ages of 90 and 83 respectively were far beyond the average of the time. As they had

---

[11] Sillers, J. (2017, July 19). *Why more ambitious goals are more likely to help*. The Orange Dot.

already lived to around 30 to 40 years old by 1776, a typical life expectancy for them was around 68 years old[12][13]. Their willingness to see a country develop into the future, I'm sure, was a key reason for them to live so long.

Having a goal on its own, however, is not enough. Indeed, there are huge benefits to vision and goal-setting but, for me, the process of working towards achieving the goal is where the real reward lies. I know from experience how the achievement of a goal can lose its novelty quite quickly, especially if we set it in the spirit of 'I will be happy when I achieve XYZ' and the feeling of happiness doesn't flow forth as soon as the goal is achieved. I truly believe the real value in goal-setting is the process or system one establishes to work towards achieving the goal. As James Clear discusses in his very popular book *Atomic Habits*, it isn't just having a goal that is important, it's the process or system we employ to achieve the goal which separates goal-achievers from the non-goal-achievers.[14]

Clear argues that there are reasons to be cautious about focusing too heavily on the goal-setting, as opposed to the process or system of achieving them. He says that "winners and losers have the same goals", so it isn't the fact the goal is there to begin with that propels a winner to the finish line first. Losers had the same goals but for whatever reason, didn't achieve them. Take, for example, the annual boat race between the Universities of Oxford and Cambridge. Those who win are ecstatic, while those who lose are absolutely crushed, emotionally and physically. Both teams shared the same goal of winning that race on that day. But the chances are, the losing team didn't employ the best process or was as relentless in adhering to it, as the winning team.

Clear's advice here, that I echo, is to "fall in love with the process rather than the product". The key is to not allow the achievement of the goal to become the only focal point; the real benefits come from

---

[12] Infoplease. (2020, August 5). *Life Expectancy by Age, 1850-2011.*

[13] Frost, N. (2018, September 4). *Two Presidents Died on the Same July 4: Coincidence or Something More?* HISTORY.

[14] Clear, J. (2020, February 4). *Forget About Setting Goals. Focus on This Instead.* James Clear.

the systems we establish. As Clear puts it: "It's not about any single accomplishment. It is about the cycle of endless refinement and continuous improvement."

I would add to this the consideration of finding happiness in the moment – in 'doing' the process or the system. If the system you employ to achieve the goal isn't enjoyable, a) the temptation to resist doing the work needed will be considerable, and b) it will make you unhappy, which could lead to resentment and the growth of a negative mindset in relation to the goal you are aiming to achieve. For example, if your goal is to lose weight, and the system you choose is an extremely restrictive diet coupled with a gruelling workout you dread, the chances are you will find any excuse to 'start tomorrow' or find a reason – any reason – why you can't make it to the gym. It's really important that the system or process you choose is enjoyable in itself, as that will increase the chances of you sticking to it and getting closer to achieving your goal. Devise a system that fits into your lifestyle, that enhances it, that makes you feel good *now*. If need be, start with something small. If your goal is to lose weight, start by getting into the habit of drinking eight glasses of water each day, which can help to clear out toxins and keep you filled up so you can snack less.

You might be thinking, how do I set my goals? Where do I begin? Below are some questions you can ask yourself to help understand what you want out of life[15]:

- Why is it that you do what you do?
- If you could do anything, what would it be?
- When was the last time you really enjoyed something and what was it?
- What thrills you (or not) about your current job role or career?
- What does a great day look like?
- What can you do today that will make your life better tomorrow?
- What did you love doing as a child? Do those things still bring you joy?

---

[15] Zupanic, M. (2019, September 20). *How To Find Your Passion*. Goalcast.

- How could you make sure you have a great day every day? What would need to happen?
- What does success look like beyond the money you earn?
- How do you want to feel about your impact on the world when and if you retire? What mark do you want to leave? How do you want to be remembered?

In the context of the purpose of this book, which is to encourage you to feel differently – more positively – about your longevity and your lifespan, I would urge you to consider setting goals and devising systems that make you feel good about yourself every single day. The better you feel about yourself, the more you love yourself now, the more positive you will feel generally, and the more resilient you will become to the challenges that life throws at you. It follows that you will be able to weather health challenges that may come your way, and they may be fewer due to your more positive outlook. This, in turn, can extend your lifespan.

Similar to the first chapter, when setting your goals,

1. Do something to make yourself happier today than you were yesterday
2. Practice a positive affirmation
3. Nourish yourself, move your body, and then rest your mind

The better you feel about yourself, and the more you see benefits in treating yourself kindly, the greater the chances you will feel stronger, more confident, more resilient and better able to achieve the longer-term goals you want to set yourself.

Becoming healthier can begin in as small a way as feeling gratitude for being alive. Once you have mastered that as a regular habit, you can further your goals by including movement, nourishment and purposeful rest. Being and feeling healthy will give you a greater chance to achieve your other goals, as well as enrich your life by being free of aches and pains.

Think about how other people factor into your goals. Don't forget to include your relationships in your goals or systems. Relationships with others – friends, family and the community - can bring real meaning and a sense of belonging into our lives.[16]

Another goal to consider is one that relates specifically to age. Many of us have accepted that our lifespan is out of our control. And it may be. However, it's worthwhile trying to set a realistic expectation or goal, perhaps one that is much longer than you originally had in your mind. Later in this book, we can put down some numbers to this expectation.

Setting goals, in my opinion, is a fun and cathartic thing to do. Try not to focus on the things you haven't achieved yet, but instead use your goal-setting activity to really think deeply about what you want. It's amazing how we don't really know the answer to this. Take some time to discover what you truly enjoy, what you truly want out of life and form a strong idea of what that looks like, for you and the people closest to you. It's important to enjoy the process of goal-setting, but also, don't feel like you have to stick to your goals too rigidly. While it's important to have a destination to aim for, it's equally important to recognise there might be times you need to pivot or recalibrate those goals. You might find something else you enjoy more and want to devote your free time to. After all, William Blake said, "The man who never alters his opinions is like standing water, and breeds reptiles of the mind."

---

[16] Hari, J. (2019). *Lost Connections: Why You're Depressed and How to Find Hope*

CHAPTER 3:

FINDING LONGEVITY IN BLUE ZONES, BUT WHAT IS THE ROLE OF SLEEP, FASTING AND AUTOPHAGY, AND MEANINGFUL RELATIONS?

L ifestyle and habits for a healthy life are now the big focus in the mainstream press; there are ketogenic diets, low-carb diets, paleo diets, more diets than we care for to be honest. Then there's the sleep monitoring, exercise, supplements, oh the endless supplements, which all seem to be popular. There is science to support some of these hot topics, however, we haven't yet got foundational research for multifactor contributions to long life. In other words, what happens if you combine some diets with special exercise regimes? Life is complicated and the combination of different effects really matters when trying to determine what is best for a long healthy life.

Dan Buettner's research into Blue Zones is the closest we've got to determining what a combination of lifestyle factors can do for our longevity.[17]

Several years ago, Buettner teamed up with National Geographic to first of all discover which areas in the world had the highest concentration of people who live to their 90th and 100th birthdays, and secondly, to gain a deep understanding of the common factors that have influenced their longevity.

---

[17] *Blue Zones—Live Longer, Better.* (2021, May 6). Blue Zones.

So far, there have been five areas identified as Blue Zones: Sardinia in Italy; Okinawa in Japan; Nicoya in Costa Rica; Loma Linda in California; and Ikaria in Greece.

Let's take a closer look at how each Blue Zone community lives, to get a sense of the commonalities, which lead to a longer lifespan.

Sardinia, Italy

The island of Sardinia boasts the world's longest-living men. The majority of these are shepherds who've been kept physically active, outdoors, as part of their livelihood. Their diets are typically Mediterranean—high in beans, sourdough bread, and according to Buettner, a type of wine called cannonau, which "contains more flavonoids than most wines."[18]

Okinawa, Japan

These Japanese islands boast the world's longest-living women in the world. Their diet is mostly plant-based, with lots of tofu, bitter melon, and turmeric. According to Buettner, one of the key differentiators between Okinawa and other communities around the world is the notion of *ikigai*, which means to be imbued with a sense of purpose, and *moai*, to have a strong social network of lifelong friends. It seems that knowing your reason for living each day and having a strong sense of belonging contributes significantly to a longer lifespan.

Nicoya, Costa Rica

Nicoya boasts the lowest rate of middle-aged mortality, which means its people have a greater chance of living longer. The traditional diet in Nicoya is dominated by three foods: corn tortillas, black beans, and squash, complemented with tropical fruits, all year round. According to Buettner, the diet is "high in complex carbohydrates, it has all the amino acids necessary for human sustenance, it's sustainable for the land, and doesn't deplete the soil or involve slaughtering animals."

---

[18] Koroshetz, K. (2019, December 18). *The Geographic Areas Where People Live the Longest—and Clues as to Why*. Goop.

Loma Linda, California

You may be surprised to learn of a Blue Zone in America—the land of burgers and fries—but Loma Linda in California is one of them. The community here belongs to members of the Seventh-Day Adventist Church, who are the longest-living Americans. Their diet is heavily influenced by the Bible, and it is largely plant-based and typically vegetarian. They have a close social network and tend to live healthier lifestyles eschewing nicotine and alcohol.

Ikaria, Greece

In Ikaria, people live about eight years longer than the average American, and there are very few cases of dementia. Their diet is typically Mediterranean, consisting of fruits and vegetables, whole grains, beans and olive oil, and according to Buettner, they also drink a lot of herbal teas with sage, oregano, and rosemary. He goes on to say that many of the greens Ikarians eat "have ten times the antioxidants you'd find in wine. And our study found that eating about half a cup of cooked greens a day is associated with about four extra years of life expectancy."

Blue Zone Diet

As you've seen from the overviews above, one of the factors in the longevity of individuals in these communities is diet. The four prevalent food groups are beans, grains, greens and nuts. In an interview with *Goop*, the holistic wellness business founded by Gwyneth Paltrow, Buettner stated that "95 to 100 percent of [the communities'] dietary intake came from low- or non-processed, plant-based food." He went so far as to say, "Unless you have an allergy or another complicating condition, most of us should be eating those four things every day. And if you are eating them, you're probably adding five years to your life expectancy."[19]

Notice that meat, fish and dairy do not factor as dominant groups. The researchers found that, on average, people in these Blue Zones eat meat around five times a month, and fish maybe twice a week.

---

[19] Koroshetz, K. (2019, December 18). *The Geographic Areas Where People Live the Longest—and Clues as to Why*. Goop.

Dairy consumption varied across the Zones but where it does feature, it is locally cultivated from animals such as sheep and goats in their care. Each community relies heavily on locally grown produce, utilising what is close to them and is more easily cultivated in their geographical environment. Sugar is also noticeably absent from many of these diets, with sweetness coming from local ingredients such as honey and herbs. And, driven by religious or spiritual traditions, intermittent fasting also becomes a way to lower blood cholesterol and trigger regenerative body processes.

Scientists have found that fasting for 12-24 hours or more triggers something called 'autophagy'. It is this which is thought to be one of the reasons why fasting is associated with longevity. Fasting is said to improve blood sugar control, reduce inflammation, encourage weight loss, and improve brain function. When we fast, or 'starve' the body for short periods of time, our cells break down proteins and other cell components and use them for energy. During autophagy, cells destroy viruses and bacteria and rid; the body of damaged structures. Japanese cell biologist, and Nobel Prize winner, Yoshinori Ohsumi famously researched autophagy and how it works. He discovered that autophagy genes are used by many species and that mutations in these genes can cause disease. Animals, plants, and single-cell organisms rely on autophagy to withstand famines. Ohsumi also showed that autophagy has a role to play in protecting the body against inflammation and the development of diseases like dementia and Parkinson's.[20]

While diet has been largely focused on in this research, mainly because of its stark differences to the meat-based diet, there were other factors found that contribute equally to a longer lifespan.

Physical movement

Interestingly, this particular research points not to rigorous cardiovascular exercise or strength-building, but to a slower, more

---

[20] Kotifani, A. (2020, June 2). *Fasting for Health and Longevity: Nobel Prize Winning Research on Cell Ageing*. Blue Zones.

purposeful movement that comes about naturally, to achieve a goal. For example, walking across fields with cattle, or gardening to grow fresh fruit and vegetables. Interestingly, the physical exercise carried out within these communities relates to everyday work and livelihood, as opposed to specific attempts to 'get fit'. Instead, physical activity forms a natural part of their lifestyle.

Having a purpose

Researchers found that a commonality in each of the Blue Zones was a confident knowledge among individuals of why they wake up in the morning. According to Buettner, "Knowing your sense of purpose is worth up to seven years of extra life expectancy." Similar to having goals, it is reassuring to understand what you want to achieve with your life – whether that is to raise children and grandchildren successfully, to do some charitable good in the world, or to simply get through each day knowing you have done the best you could.

Slow the pace

We're all familiar with the consequences of a stressful lifestyle. Stress doesn't only come from having a high-pressured, desk job with endless 24hr emails; stress can be caused by a family argument, or scarcity of resources. The difference with the Blue Zone communities is in the way they actively seek to reduce stress or manage it, whether that's through taking a moment to be mindful or to pray, take a nap or enjoy social time with a glass of wine.

The 80% rule

Another commonality among the communities is a mindfulness about when to eat and when to stop eating. For many individuals, the smallest meal is eaten at the end of the day, and they stop eating when their stomachs are 80% full, to avoid weight gain.

Alcohol

Somewhat surprisingly, researchers found that drinking alcohol moderately and regularly can contribute to longevity. According to Buettner, "Moderate drinkers outlive non-drinkers. The trick is to drink 1-2 glasses per day, with friends and/or with food."

Sense of belonging

The feeling of being part of a community is very important in achieving longevity. In the Blue Zones, communities tended to be faith-based, attending regular services. This, according to Buettner, "will add 4-14 years of life expectancy." The company you keep can have a lasting effect on your state of mind and your longevity. Blue Zone researchers found that the networks of longer-living people played a key role in shaping their health behaviours.

Families first

It is common for people living in Blue Zones to keep their families close, often having ageing grandparents live in the home, alongside grandchildren. This is said to lower disease and mortality rates of children in the home, too. Furthermore, committing to a life partner can add up to 3 years of life expectancy.

Sleep

Another factor is sleep. It has been widely reported that for optimal performance during the day, humans require eight hours of sleep every night, but we've all heard stories about high-profile successful people who manage to thrive on four or five hours instead. It is argued that a lengthier sleep on a regular basis can reduce the risk of serious diseases including Alzheimer's and various cancers. Blue Zones show that the people who do make it to their 100th birthday get sufficient sleep, meaning 8-10 hours a day. This could come as a bit of shock, but even 6 or 7 hours is detrimental in the long run.

While there hasn't been a huge amount of research in longevity in this area, some very interesting observations have been made by the sleep expert Matthew Walker in his enlightening book, Why We Sleep.[21] Walker is the Director of the Centre for Human Sleep Science at the University of California, Berkeley. In his book, he reports that, "Routinely sleeping less than six or seven hours a night demolishes your immune system, more than doubling your risk of cancer. Insufficient sleep is a key lifestyle factor determining whether or not you will develop Alzheimer's disease."

---

[21] Walker, M. (2018). *Why We Sleep: Unlocking the Power of Sleep and Dreams.*

Walker goes on to cite a study by Dr Michael Irwin at the University
of California, Los Angeles, who conducted research into the impact
of sleep on cancer-fighting immune cells. "Examining healthy young
men, Irwin demonstrated that a single night of four hours of sleep –
such as going to bed at three a.m. and waking up at seven a.m. –
swept away 70 percent of the natural killer cells circulating in the
immune system, relative to a full eight-hour night of sleep."[22] We
simply need to have a long night's sleep to maintain our immune
system.

Walker also references the impact of sleep on other physical and
psychological factors. According to his research, even a moderate
reduction in sleep for one week can disrupt blood sugar levels to the
point of pre-diabetic status. And he further asserts that sleep
disruption also contributes to all major psychiatric conditions,
including depression, anxiety and suicidality.[23]

A report by the Sleep Foundation echoes this, stating that, "In adults,
a lack of sleep has been associated with a wide range of negative
health consequences including cardiovascular problems, a weakened
immune system, higher risk of obesity and type II diabetes, impaired
thinking and memory, and mental health problems like depression
and anxiety." The report goes on to say, "These diverse ramifications
of sleep deprivation offer strong support to the view that sleep
doesn't have just one biological purpose but in fact, through its
complexity, is an important contributor to the proper functioning of
nearly all of the systems of the body."[24]

To finish, one pertinent conclusion that Walker draws, is "the shorter
you sleep, the shorter your life span." It seems to be the case that one
very clear way to increase your longevity is to get at least eight hours
of sleep every night.

[22] Four Pillar Freedom. (2019, November 13). *Why We Sleep by Matthew Walker: Summary and Notes*.
[23] Four Pillar Freedom. (2019, November 13). *Why We Sleep by Matthew Walker: Summary and Notes*.
[24] Suni, E. (2020, October 23). *How Sleep Works*. Sleep Foundation.

Make sleep work for you: Here are my top tips.

1. Stick to a sleep schedule
Give your body the best chance of settling into a sleep/wake rhythm by setting yourself a schedule every night. Aim to be in bed for a certain time and plan a routine that leads up to that time, so your body starts to learn when sleep time is approaching. And set an alarm for the same time every morning. Eventually, this may help to train your body clock so that it recognises when the window for sleep begins and ends, and before long, you may not even need an alarm.

2. Exercise earlier in the day
It's important to exercise. Getting outside in the daylight is important for regulating the body's circadian rhythms – the daily cycles of sleep and wakefulness. But exercising late in the day can energize you to the point you may find it difficult to wind down and relax before bed. Try to exercise earlier in the day if you can, even if this means just going for walk outside as the sun comes up – that could make for a powerful, beautiful, life-affirming start to the day.

3. Avoid caffeine and nicotine
Both caffeine and nicotine are stimulants that can stay in the body for long periods, potentially keeping you awake for longer, or causing disruption to your sleep. It is best to avoid these altogether, or perhaps limit yourself to one cup of a caffeinated drink in the morning. As we've seen in the diets of those who live in the Blue Zones, caffeinated drinks rarely get a mention.

4. Avoid large meals, beverages and alcoholic drinks late at night
Try to eat your final meal of the day earlier in the evening and keep the portion size fairly small. This way, your body doesn't go to bed still working hard to digest the food. If it is still hard at work, the body can't fully relax and restore itself overnight. Try to think of your food more as fuel. You need fuel to power you through your day; you don't need food to power you through sleep. It has been shown that smaller meals more often are the best way to eat for optimal health.

5. Take naps but not after 3pm

I love this tip. Who knew naps were good for you? As we learned above, napping is an accepted part of the day in some of the Blue Zone communities. Your body performs better if it can rest for a period during the day. So, if you can find the space and time to nap, go ahead, but avoid napping after 3pm as this can affect your ability to go to sleep at night.

6. Create the right atmosphere for sleep

A cool, dark room tends to be the most conducive to a good night's sleep, so if you can, try sleeping with a window open or the heaters turned off, and black-out blinds or heavy curtains over the windows. Remove all electronic gadgets from the room so that you are not tempted to use them late at night. According to the Sleep Foundation, "The blue light emitted by many devices disrupts the natural production of melatonin, a hormone that facilitates sleep and can throw off your circadian rhythm.

Pulling all these factors together

We would do well to learn from the communities who live in the Blue Zones, the lifestyles they lead and the way they look after themselves. These are all very natural, localised ways of life – in most cases, traditional for that culture. What I find particularly interesting is the importance of connection and community in the blueprint of longevity indicated by the Blue Zone lifestyles. As Buettner suggested, having these types of connections or a community-based faith could increase our life expectancy by 4-14 years. This is echoed by the US National Alliance on Mental Illness which gives the following definition of community:

"When simplified down to its most important element, community is all about connection. Community is not just an entity or a group of people, it's a feeling. It's feeling connected to others, feeling accepted for who you are and feeling supported. Having connection can help us feel wanted and loved." [25] When people feel valued and supported, their health reaps benefits. When our health status improves, the less likely we are to suffer from illness and disease, and our life expectancy can be increased.

The conveniences we have nowadays – the supermarkets that stock everything we could possibly wish for, and the light relief of Netflix or movies after your working day – make it very tempting to move away from some of the more natural ways of living that have resulted in longevity in those Blue Zones. It takes discipline to adopt a new, simpler lifestyle. But I hope the findings above persuade you to try, if only with a little step at a time. The benefits you could reap are profound.

[25] Gilbert, S. (2019, November 18). *The Importance of Community and Mental Health / NAMI: National Alliance on Mental Illness*. NAMI: National Alliance on Mental Illness.

CHAPTER 4:

HOW TO EXTEND YOUR LIFE LIKE A BILLIONAIRE

There has been a huge amount of progress in terms of scientific discovery and understanding when it comes to increasing our longevity and maintaining health. There are a myriad of ways in which we could potentially add years to our lives, not only by learning from Blue Zones, but also by taking advantage of therapies and services that are now available. As with most innovations, they are often costly to the consumer at first, but as technology advances and competitors enter the marketplace, costs come down and the same services and products become affordable to more people. Most of these are already surprisingly affordable, especially when compared against end-of-life healthcare that we typically incur.

We will look at some of those innovations currently available for those who can afford them. If you are fortunate enough to have unlimited resources or even some disposable income for your health, then there are quite a few compelling options.

There are a few key areas though where the very wealthy spend their money to increase their healthspan. After a lot of research, it seems to me that it's concentrated in the following categories:

1. Selfie: Medical monitoring including gene mapping of their DNA and microbiome. This provides bespoke knowledge for both lifestyle and medical healthcare
2. Remedy: Medical healthcare to treat diseases early in their development
3. Reverse: Rejuvenation therapies
4. Help: Services and technology to aid exercise and a healthy lifestyle

We'll now go through each of these areas in more detail.

One idea to start with is that if you can treat it, then get it sorted. And crucially, we now have the technology to find out what is wrong with us really early on. We can scan and find diseases when we know there is something wrong with us, or we can scan ourselves regularly to see ongoing changes and prevent things from making us ill in the future.

Selfie: Understanding your baseline health now

One theory we are all familiar with is that knowledge is power and knowing the current state of our health truly does empower us to use the information and take steps towards creating a healthier future for ourselves.

For a few years, healthcare providers have been offering a suite of tests that will diagnose a person's current state of health. These can be as simple as testing for blood pressure, digestive health and cholesterol levels, or they can go deeper into exploring for possible early signs of cancer and heart disease by carrying out various tests on blood samples. As you can imagine, the notion of testing for present and future health has continued to advance, and with some investment, you can undergo a six month or annual full body scan and testing regime. These scans could help you to better understand your genetic make-up through genomic sequencing and the state of your gut bacteria (microbiome), and even the proteins in your body (proteomics), which can determine the health of your cells and their ability to repair themselves. Of course, some services will also put your body through an MRI scanner to identify any issues within the organs and structure of your body.

In 2018, one of these healthcare providers, Human Longevity, published data on the test results of its first 1,190 clients, to demonstrate the benefits of conducting such tests in terms of acquiring valuable knowledge:
- 2% of patients had undiagnosed tumours or advanced cancer

- 2.5% of patients had undiagnosed aneurysms, which is very high on the list of diseases that can kill you
- 9% of patients had previously undetected coronary artery disease (coronary heart disease is the most common cause of death in the world)
- In total, 14.4% had significant issues requiring immediate intervention, while 40% percent found a condition that needed long-term monitoring[26]

If those clients hadn't undergone the suite of tests, they may not have known about the risks to their health until it was too late. This clearly demonstrates the benefits of acquiring knowledge that can empower us to make the changes we need to, to increase our lifespan.

Bestselling author, entrepreneur and founder of X-Prize, Peter Diamandis is a convert to 'selfie' medical testing. It's a large part of his coaching program, and on his website, he states: "The test measures your biological age, mitochondrial health, immune health, gut microbiome, cellular health, and 30 other health scores. It also makes recommendations on what foods and supplements you should target to reduce inflammation and reverse your biological age with the goal of giving you more energy, boosting immunity, better gut and mental health, on the path to a longer, healthier life."[27]

The idea of these tests as 'selfies' has been taken, very literally, to the point at which we can now take a 'selfie' using a phone camera and the result is a medical diagnosis of some kind.

A study by the American Heart Association, reports on a "new technology called transdermal optical imaging that measures blood pressure continuously and without contact from video of a person's face." The research showed that, although there was still room for improvement to the usability, "this technology exhibits comparable accuracy to traditional automated blood pressure monitors."

[26] Diamandis, P. H. (2020, October 18). *Increase your healthspan, now*. Diamandis.
[27] Diamandis, P. H. (2020, October 18). *Increase your healthspan, now*. Diamandis.

We need to understand our own genetic picture as this arms us with information about potential health issues we could be treating now, as well as conditions we may be susceptible to in the future. It is most useful to do this on an ongoing basis as this way, you are more likely to notice changes that might be taking place within your body that could be better improved with early treatment or intervention. Having greater knowledge of your health status will help you to better plan your future. You may consider yourself to be in good health even if you have certain medical conditions such as high blood pressure or osteoarthritis. You may feel well in yourself while unknowingly developing a chronic, progressive, ultimately fatal illness such as Alzheimer's or metastatic colon cancer.[28] Knowing what the reality is when it comes to your current and possible future state of health puts you in the powerful position of being able to create goals that support your health and therefore your longevity.

Remedy diseases as early as possible

The ultra-wealthy use the same drugs and procedures that you find in most modern hospitals, although the care and rehabilitation may feel like five-star luxury. You have access to many of the same treatments so there really is no reason not to understand what your body needs to help heal, so you can look forward to a longer and healthier life.

Keep your vitamins topped up. Supplements are very popular, but it seems to be a complicated area with lots of advice. Diet-based research is discussed more commonly amongst scientists. The most supported supplements are your daily vitamins, such as Vitamin A, B6, C, D and E and Zinc as recommended by your medical practitioner.

There is much more to discuss regarding diet to support healthy processes in our bodies. To look at the research in more detail, we will review diets and fasting in chapter 7.

---

[28] Harvard Health. (2020, June 17). *Understanding your health status.*

Reverse ageing with rejuvenation therapies

Regeneration

Anti-ageing has been a buzzword for many years, and products that claim to halt or reverse the ageing process, whether they have been scientifically proven or not, are in high demand. No longer confined to cosmetic products, the notion of anti-ageing or 'turning back the clock' is a prevalent topic in scientific research. Scientific labs across the world have some of the leading minds in all of biological research focusing on tests that literally make our cells young. We are talking about altering DNA, manipulating our cell's primal functions, decoding the interlacing epigenetic codes that control ageing. All of this is happening right now and will lead to lifespan altering improvements within the next decade. Before we get into that, let's look at what has been around for a while already.

There are many approaches to slowing down the ageing process, now available to people who can afford them.

We will look at the science and how people are using breakthroughs in research in chapter 6 and chapter 8.

Stem cell regeneration

Regenerative medicine is a type of medicine that uses stem cells to repair tissues that have been damaged. Stem cells are undifferentiated cells, cells that are not yet determined for a specific function, that can transform into other specialized cells. Doctors can harvest stem cells from the human body and then use them to reconstruct damaged tissue.

As we age, our supply of stem cells declines in quality and quantity. It's for this reason, alternative sources of stem cells are increasingly being explored. Organs that are well-known sources of stem cells are the placenta and umbilical cord. The stem cells within these organs have been found to help reduce inflammation and repair joints. They can also fight autoimmune diseases and restore organ functionality.

Scientists at the Albert Einstein College of Medicine, New York, found that the lives of mice could be extended by 10-15% when stem cells were injected into their brains. This finding has positive implications for the development of further anti-ageing therapies in humans.[29]

We will look at stem cell science in more detail in chapter 9.

Young blood

It is possible now to purchase a blood transfusion using the blood of a younger person, to—supposedly—literally, pump you full of youth. The benefits of this practice haven't yet been widely proven but there are some high profile converts to this practice, including billionaire PayPal co-founder-turned-venture capitalist, Peter Thiel.[30]

Help: Services and technology to aid exercise and a healthy lifestyle

Light therapy

It is reasonably well-known that white light can be used to treat Seasonal Affective Disorder (SAD), but other forms of light are now gaining in popularity thanks to the recognition of their benefits in rejuvenating different parts of our bodies.

According to a report in the US National Library of Medicine, there is increasing evidence to suggest that light can play an important role in the regulation of ageing and longevity. While Ultra-violet (UV) radiation causes cells' genetic code to degrade and therefore harm our bodies, Near-Infrared (NIR) light is thought to show protective effects. There are a number of possible beneficial uses for visible light

---

[29] Hildreth, C. (2020, October 12). *Can We Extend the Human Lifespan With Regenerative Medicine?* BioInformant.
[30] Finance, A. (2020, May 22). *How Billionaires Plan to Live Forever | ABC Finance Ltd.* ABC Finance.

including circadian rhythm control, the inducing of oxidative stress, and retinal activity to affect neuronal circuits and systems.[31]

Light therapy has been recognised as being beneficial for treating neurodegenerative disorders, Alzheimer's and Parkinson's disease. These two diseases develop as the result of a progressive death of many neurons in the brain, a crippling and horrendous outcome as all too many of us have had an experience of. As reported in the US National Library of Medicine, Red to Infrared light therapy, and in particular light in the Near Infrared range, is emerging as a safe and effective therapy that is capable of arresting neuronal death.[32] As we learn more about these effects, we can combine the findings with other scientific breakthroughs in understanding our brain function decline.

Exercise as prevention

This theme is more accessible and perhaps more familiar to most people. There have already been significant advances in technology that enable us to monitor our exercise and some of our physiological health factors such as blood pressure. Many people already use phone apps and smart watches to track these factors throughout the day, and there are exercise machines like Peloton that will tailor specific exercise programs to meet the needs of different individuals.

There has, however, been further advancements in technology that the very wealthy are already taking advantage of. Companies such as Vasper, CAROL Bike, and Kaatsu use artificial intelligence to better map your exercise programs to your particular situation. They may also use compression bands and cooling temperatures to adjust your body's reaction to the training, which can make the workouts more intense and can also help to aid recovery.

And after all that exercise, there is now a Magnetic Resonance Pad which is designed to help the individual relax and unwind at the end

---

[31] Shen, J. (2019, May 30). *Effects of light on ageing and longevity.* PubMed.
[32] Johnstone, D. (2016, January 11). *Turning On Lights to Stop Neurodegeneration: The Potential of Near Infrared Light Therapy in Alzheimer's and Parkinson's Disease.* PubMed Central (PMC).

of the day by resetting your body's magnetism. It is argued that this can help to provide a better night's sleep.[33]

There are so many exciting technologies being developed to make our exercise more effective. And they all look fun to try and may make you feel better. They'll certainly be conversation starters with your friends. But we know for sure that some exercise every week will be beneficial for the long-term. After discussing the science of ageing in chapter 5, we will revisit some science about exercise in chapter 7.

The last hurrah - happily ever after

It's all well and good being able to extend your life now, and rejuvenate yourself as much as you can afford, but what if your true goal is everlasting life? Well, what do you know? There are now options for that too.

Freezing the human body for later resurrection might be the subject of many a sci-fi Hollywood movie, but there are now companies such as Alcor Life Extension Foundation, Cryonics Institute, Suspended Animation Inc. and KrioRus, that will freeze parts of or the whole of your body. The idea is to 'reanimate' the body once the medical community has discovered cures to various diseases or solutions to halt the ageing process. However, the results of this haven't been proven and it is largely viewed as pseudo-science.[34]

If you're more concerned about preserving your brain as opposed to your body, you could now look into Digital Consciousness. This may sound like yet another sci-fi movie but when highly regarded institutions like MIT and the US National Institute of Medical Health

---

[33] Casaroma Wellness. (2021, January 13). *The iMRS - Pulsed Magnetic Resonance Stimulation Mat.*
[34] Finance, A. (2020, May 22). *How Billionaires Plan to Live Forever | ABC Finance Ltd.* ABC Finance.

start pumping huge amounts of money into research of memory it's worth being aware of.[35]

Life is becoming more complex, and we've looked at a few areas that the very wealthy are attracted to improve their health and lifespan. It's necessary to now go into a bit of science to understand what ageing is and how we can harness this knowledge into actionable improvements for our day to day lives. If some of the unusual things covered in this chapter have put you off, then in later chapters you may find information about diet and alternative medicine is far more interesting. However, in the meantime, we can get into the science and where astounding breakthroughs are being made in healthcare.

---

[35] Finance, A. (2020, May 22). *How Billionaires Plan to Live Forever | ABC Finance Ltd*. ABC Finance.

CHAPTER 5:

AGEING IS A DISEASE - THEORY OR FACT?

D o we get diseases due to ageing, or is ageing a treatable disease in itself? Is heart disease the same as ageing? Can we cure ageing, and never get Alzheimer's? These are intricate questions and experts are only starting to discuss them openly. It will soon become better understood, but for the time being, this is still open for discussion.

According to David Sinclair, a leading geneticist professor based at Harvard Medical School, "Medicine should view ageing not as a natural consequence of growing older, but as a condition in and of itself." As concluded by the MIT Technology Review, which published Sinclair's quote, "Old age, in his view, is simply a pathology—and, like all pathologies, can be successfully treated", then the labelling of age is important. If ageing can be labelled a disease, and you can die of old age, then funding and research will flourish in the methods to tackle ageing. There is progress building in this area, as the category formally used across history is starting to make a comeback. The definition of a disease affecting less than half of a population certainly inhibited progress, this is starting to be acknowledged as not fit for purpose as scientists unearth more and more signs of specific ageing processes in our bodies that can be modified, improved and reversed.[36]

Whether you agree with these statements or not, this is a very real question now being debated by experts in this field.

---

[36] Adam, D. (2021, April 30). *What if ageing weren't inevitable, but a curable disease?* MIT Technology Review.

How do we measure ageing?

There have been significant technological developments in this area that allow us to understand how we define age (here is a clue: it doesn't always have to be calculated by 'years' since birth), and then determine how old our bodies are, biologically speaking.

Biomarkers are biological measures of a biological state, and they can be used to identify our biological age. They are often used in clinical assessments for blood pressure or cholesterol levels and can be used to monitor and predict a person's health status so that appropriate treatment can be arranged.

There are several different biomarkers in use today, for measuring the likes of cardiovascular systems, metabolic systems and immune systems. They are generally easy to use and effective, for that reason they are routinely used in medical examinations.

The results of these biomarkers can tell us different things about the state of our health in many areas. If we are generally fit and healthy for our age, for example, biomarkers may suggest we are physiologically younger than our years suggest.

As the body ages, changes take place gradually and over a long time so, at any given stage, those changes appear to be modest. Changes can be shifts in the populations of bacteria that live in our gut (our microbiome) to differences in our DNA. Specifically for that latter biomarker, there are natural changes in our DNA over time, whereby the levels of DNA methylation (a change that occurs to our DNA molecules) can be measured to provide an epigenetic clock for our bodies.

Scientists are concluding that there are many changes that lead to ageing: dysfunction of our energy systems, mitochondria; genomic instability that causes DNA damage; telomere shortening; epigenome alterations (the control systems of our DNA); loss of proteostasis to control the use of proteins; deregulated nutrient sensing; accumulation of senescent cells; stem cell exhaustion; altered intercellular communication; and the production of inflammatory molecules. All of these changes build up, sometimes cumulatively, to make it far harder for our body to function healthily. This will lead to other diseases forming, which we call 'age-related' diseases such as ones we are too commonly aware of, such as cardiovascular disease, cancer, arthritis, or osteoporosis. It's hard even to write down these diseases without finding the trauma of such things overwhelming. But the very fact that I can write down that scientists know about the finer details of ageing is the most amazing silver lining. Although I won't cover all of the ageing changes in this book, I will cover some in enough detail for you to see progress in minimising ageing.

Each of the changes that lead to ageing can be addressed scientifically, and there are some of the finest health and medical experts working on finding solutions to each of these. It is very exciting to think that these problems are likely to be solved, and we will benefit from the science to massively increase our health into old age.

Not only can we look to science to intervene, but as we adjust our bodies with better simple habits, our biological age can become younger, and so a 60-year-old can quite easily have the body of a 48-year-old for example, or younger. As we get older, we still think of ourselves as much younger. As the build-up of good practice and technology combine, soon we may have the neuron health of a younger brain too.

Perhaps the science is only starting to catch up with what people have been assured of for years. The 76-year-old Michel de Carvalho, chairman of private wealth manager Capital Generation Partners, described his personal method, "A man has three ages – the one stamped on his passport, his biological age and finally his mental age. 'You blend the three together and divide by three and you come up with your actual age. So I'm about 47,' he states. 'Massively helped by my mental age'".[37]

---

[37] Marsh, A. (2021, May 24). *Olympian, actor. . . wealth manager? Meet Michel de Carvalho, one half of Britain's ninth richest couple.* Spear's Magazine.

The role of telomeres and senescent cells in the ageing process

There are many theories within the scientific community regarding the questions of why and how we age. One that has dominated the discussion in recent years centres on the subject of telomeres. These are little protective caps at the ends of the DNA molecules that make up our chromosomes (if you remember high-school biology, the chromosomes in the nucleus are where our DNA information is stored). Telomeres' job is to stop the ends of chromosomes from fraying, much like the plastic tips on the ends of shoelaces.[38]

When our cells divide, telomeres ensure our DNA is copied properly. Normally, with each cell division, some of the DNA information (nucleotides) is left out, leading to some loss of genetic information. As telomeres lose information, they become shorter during the process of cell division.

Telomeres are the reason our cells still contain DNA. They consist of the same nucleotides repeated again and again, so even though the telomeres get shorter over time, they can still protect the rest of the DNA.

It is thought that the shortening of telomeres is one of the factors which causes cells to age. When telomeres are too short, a cell can no longer divide. There is a limit for the natural number of times a cell divides, and this limit has been named after Leonard Hayflick.[39] The Hayflick limit is about 50 cell divisions. And, when a telomere structure becomes too short, our cells stop replicating. At this point, the cell becomes inactive, or 'senescent'. An inactive cell then dies and is cleared by our body; this prevents injured or even cancerous cells from spreading, thus containing any damage within our bodies.

Another area of science that leads to ageing, is the accumulation of senescent cells due to telomere shortening. Senescent cells are when the natural process of a cell dying doesn't work. Instead, the cell that

---

[38] Australian Academy of Science, & Graves, J. (2018, October 10). *What are telomeres?* Australian Academy of Science.
[39] Shay, J. W. (2000, October 1). *Hayflick, his limit, and cellular ageing.* Nature Reviews Molecular Cell Biology.

should be cleared away just remains and doesn't function properly. Senescent cells can be problematic.

According to James Kirkland, a researcher for the Mayo Clinic, specialising in cellular senescence, "It's very hard to kill [senescent cells]. If you grow them under conditions that would kill a normal cell, they'll survive and sometimes survive for years under those conditions."[40]

In some cases, these senescent cells can start to impact our normal tissue function, particularly because they create inflammation which is then linked to cellular ageing. As we get older, senescent cells begin to build up in greater amounts in our bodies, accelerating the process of ageing. Scientists now believe that this build-up might be a factor in conditions such as arthritis, diabetes and cardiovascular disease.

Aside from the ageing aspect, senescent cells can be good for us. These cells are fundamentally protective for certain conditions, such as when a cell realises it is too damaged to continue. Early on, senescent cells help control the growth of tissue in embryos. Later on in our lives, senescent cells help wound repair. Also, if a cell develops a cancerous mutation and begins to divide uncontrollably to form a tumour, a cell might go senescent to prevent further multiplication. Nonetheless, we are finding that there is merit to do something about the *build-up* of senescent cells.

Is there a way to helpfully clear these senescent cells though? Yes. Firstly, our body does this naturally; sometimes though old cells just don't get cleared. We are finding ways to help clear senescent cells and there are drugs or even topical creams in the field of senolytics. This may be an exciting new area for anti-ageing cosmetics. And who knows where these scientific studies and products will lead.

Early studies have shown that senolytic treatments, designed to remove senescent cells, could help us combat old age. In a 2019 study, James Kirkland gave a small group of diabetic kidney patients

---

[40] Scharping, N. (2020, August 11). *Senolytics: A New Weapon in the War on Ageing.* Discover Magazine.

senolytic drugs for three days. Follow-ups indicated that the number of senescent cells in their bodies had been reduced, which indicated there was merit in further exploring the use of such medication for treating age-related disease.[41]

Treating senescent cells is the burgeoning field of "senolytic" drugs. Investments in these areas are where you find billionaire household names such as Amazon founder Jeff Bezos and PayPal cofounder Peter Thiel, who we have already mentioned is investing in regenerative medicine.

Working with telomeres

While there is no strong correlation between lifespan and initial telomere length, a strong correlation has been found between lifespan and telomere shortening *rate*.[42]

There are ways now in which we can act to lengthen our telomeres, which can prolong the life of our cells and reduce the number that become senescent to begin with. Lifestyle is an important determinant of telomere length.

According to US healthcare provider, Daisy Health, there are five key ways we can adopt a telomere-friendly lifestyle:

1. Maintain a healthy weight

Obesity is a factor in many serious health issues, including diabetes and heart disease. Research has found obesity can indicate shorter telomeres. According to the article, "The loss of telomeres in obese individuals is the equivalent to 8.8 years of life" therefore a dramatic shortening of lifespan.

---

[41] Scharping, N. (2020, August 11). *Senolytics: A New Weapon in the War on Ageing.* Discover Magazine.
[42] Whittemore, K. (2019, July 23). *Telomere shortening rate predicts species life span.* PNAS.

2. Exercise regularly

Research has shown that exercise can reduce oxidative stress, which is known to impact cell function and therefore DNA. According to their research, one study found that "men in their 50s who were active runners had nearly the same telomere length as men in their 20s". Cardiovascular exercise of any type, so long as not utterly destructive, seems to help.

3. Manage chronic stress

It is suspected that stress can contribute to telomere shortening, as people who "face adversity early in life and those who are burdened by chronic caregiving, heavy workloads and financial stress, have shorter telomeres than others." These are broad-brush indicators of chronic stress, but it doesn't mean avoiding those types of caregiving jobs. Perhaps those that were able to have a positive mindset towards their stressful workloads or financial issues, would not have suffered from shortened telomeres. Granted, it would take extra special mental effort to overcome obviously difficult situations.

4. Eat a telomere-protective diet

It is possible to maintain your telomeres through a healthy and nutritious wholefood diet. Prioritise foods that are high in vitamin C and antioxidants such as fresh fruit and vegetables, whole grains and plant-based protein. Aim to reduce or avoid red and processed meats, sodium, sugar, caffeine and large volumes of alcohol, which all seem to have a mildly negative effect in generating more stress in our digestive system and fundamental biological processes.

All that being said, science has found that telomeres have a key function, and altering them too much can cause problems. We have to be careful not to over-lengthen our telomeres through drastic medical interventions because the shortening of telomeres performs a critical function.

If a telomere becomes too short, it very cleverly sends a signal to the rest of the cell that there's a problem with the DNA and it needs to be repaired by cellular repair mechanisms. In this way, telomeres play a highly important role in preventing cellular disease such as cancer, which is, in effect, a state where cell division is uncontrolled. If we only focused on lengthening our telomeres in a bid to slow down the ageing process, we could be compromising their ability to prevent cancers.

Radical energy and ageing

In addition to the shortening of telomeres and the sometimes-destructive existence of senescent cells, the very energy system of our body seems to also be a cause of ageing.

Mitochondria is the life-giving, energy machine within our cells and can generate reactive oxygen species (ROS) that damage both mitochondrial and nuclear genomes (DNA), thereby increasing the likelihood of senescent cells forming. The production of ROS is thought to increase with age. This makes antioxidants in our diet potentially even more important in terms of prolonging our natural life, because these antioxidants can sweep away all the debris ROS from our mitochondria energy processes.

Smoking cigarettes is a known cause of ROS, and it adds to the cellular stress within our bodies. Poor quality air – air impacted by pollution – can have the same effect.

Not only does ROS impact our DNA, but they can also damage the structure of our cells and our hormones, altering the way in which they can function. A large number of studies have linked ROS to smoking and poor air quality, as well as to cancer and respiratory, neurodegenerative and digestive diseases. And yet naturally produced ROS is a part of life, so as long as we maintain low levels of ROS by avoiding smoking, then our natural body functions, along with potentially adding antioxidants into our diet, can keep us in good condition.

In summary

We now have tools that can measure our physiological age to determine if we are ageing slower or faster than the years since birth. There are many factors in ageing, that when combined give us a very useful picture of our bodies and the likelihood of age-related diseases. We also know a rapid shortening or breakage in telomeres can lead to increased numbers of senescent cells. There are simple habits that can keep these telomeres at their natural length, and most of these habits are common amongst people living to a very old age in Blue Zones. The top four factors are exercise, a healthy diet including plenty of antioxidants, lower stress levels, and avoiding smoking.

There are mixed views about calling ageing a disease. The proponents believe it is important to label ageing as a disease to bring in funding and research to combat the ageing process. People who oppose this believe that labels of ageing disease hurt society by applying stigma to older people. Opposition also thinks that money flooding into a new anti-ageing industry will provide expensive solutions and drugs. All of this could shift attention away from people being advised to lead a healthy lifestyle, which could be far more effective. I have some sympathy for this line of argument and hope that education, such as this book will help alleviate those concerns.

Diseases are currently classified as affecting less than half of the population, while ageing clearly affects everyone. However, it seems that ageing is undoubtedly a breakdown of how our body works, and something that can be treated.

In my opinion, and I am wordsmithing the definitions, ageing is going to be called a disease, despite ageing being part of life. We don't think of life as a disease, but the dysfunction of certain processes of our bodies should be labelled as a disease. To me, it's more interesting to focus on the rate of natural ageing, and how that can be extended healthily as far as possible. Extending life by treating the signs of damage in our bodies is the way forward.

Ageing is part of life for the time being, but we already have some solutions and will find even more to slow and reverse ageing and eradicate age-related diseases.

CHAPTER 6:

WHERE ARE THINGS GOING NEXT? NEW SCIENCES AND BREAKTHROUGHS

As we've discussed, there are already quite a few ways we can understand more about the health status of our bodies and the things we can do to affect our longevity through diet, exercise, sleep patterns and stress management. Technology has developed to a point where incredibly valuable information about our health can sit in our very own hands.

Our phones, for example, track our movements in ways we couldn't have imagined a decade ago. Smart homes with voice assistants are understanding our habits, as well as determining our health status simply using the sound of our voice. The ability of an Apple Watch to recognise a fall and then call for help is truly life-enhancing.

Hopefully, the prescient health prompts and nudges provided by these large tech companies, will be led by science to be in our own interests. Luckily, so far it seems that there are highly credible institutions involved like the National Health Service in the UK, international hospital networks, many state-level US health organisations and the US National Health Association.

In this chapter, I'm going to discuss some of the ways in which technology has advanced to open up a world of possibility when it comes to better understanding and managing our health.

Big data

The benefits of big data analytics are plentiful in the healthcare industry. The vast majority of healthcare sectors and providers will reap the benefits of big data implementation within digital medicine. Hospitals, private practices and other providers will be better positioned to make even more accurate decisions, quickly, based on the data provided.

It isn't just the public and private healthcare providers that stand to benefit from the entry of big data into the healthcare sector, it's the patients and customers themselves.

In an article by social and digital consultancy experts, Linchpin, it is argued that "People want more of a say in the healthcare decision-making process, and the advances in the precision medicine field are allowing consumers the chance to give their input. The growing emphasis on consumer-based practices combined with precision medicine advances is providing increased transparency and more clarity about the costs of care of treatment."[43]

In his book, The Future is Faster than you think, Peter Diamandis defends his view that big technology companies will be running healthcare by 2030. Referencing the fact that Amazon has partnered with health providers in the UK and US to give broadly approved responses to basic health questions, such as 'how can I get rid of a cold?' There are now over 2,000 health wellness skills on its platform all using and feeding into Big Data analysis.

He notes that, similarly, Google Assistant uses search data to serve up information about medications, symptoms, and diseases, as well as providing interactions with physicians and medical services. Both the Google Home and the Echo have a Mayo Clinic-developed skill called First Aid that helps people navigate minor injuries. Apple also tackles personal health through its interconnected devices and apps. Apple's HealthKit connects to devices such as the Apple Watch which, in turn, gathers data about the user's health and fitness status.

---

[43] Ross, B. (2021, March 7). *Trends Transforming The Precision Medicine Industry In 2021 from*. Linchpin SEO.

According to Diamandis, "the more information is available about you—your genetic makeup, your health history, what you ate for breakfast, the bacteria in your bowel movement, how you slept last night, what kind of sound you're exposed to every day—the better artificial intelligence will be at spotting your potential for illness and suggesting care before the problem becomes intractable."[44]

Artificial intelligence

The pace of development of Artificial Intelligence (AI) is astounding. It's now possible for AI to recognise important patterns in our habits and movements that are going to be relevant and, dare I say it, crucial for our lifespan. As we all know, sedentary lifestyles aren't ideal for our general health, and this seriously impacts our levels of fitness and physical abilities. Sleep cycles and general sleep quality can now be measured by anyone with a smartphone, and this analysis can inform us to focus more on wind-down activities to improve our rest. But there will be subtle examples that come in the future that we wouldn't know if it weren't for AI insights.

AI in medicine will be able to exponentially improve research, improve therapies, identify optimal delivery for drugs. All of this can be bespoke for each person because we are all unique at a very detailed level. When it comes to medicine and healthcare, these differences between us can matter. Allergic reactions are serious considerations, but so are drug efficacy factors in our bodies. Getting the exact right advice and personal healthcare will be completely different to the traditional medical care that we have grown up with. Our DNA and the way that our DNA acts (epigenetic differences) mean that we all have slightly different responses to medicines and healthcare, and technology nowadays can interpret how medicine will work - in advance! We don't find this in clinics yet, but the findings are being worked into the healthcare system and before too long we will all get truly bespoke treatment.

---

[44] Reader, R. (2019, December 16). *Amazon and Apple will be our doctors in the future, says tech guru Peter Diamandis*. Fast Company.

Genomic sequencing and editing

I may have glossed over the fact that we can scan our DNA down to the very detail of each molecule. This is a mind-boggling achievement. Figuring out every 3 billion molecule pairs and their ordering is called DNA Sequencing. Sequencing can be done cheaply now. Originally, the cost of sequencing was $100 million per genome, and it is now far cheaper; to below $1,000 per genome (current estimates are as low as a few hundred dollars). What is potentially more fascinating is that we can do things with our DNA molecules at such fine detail, which is called gene therapy or gene editing.

Genome editing is described by the National Human Genome Association as "a method that lets scientists change the DNA of many organisms, including plants, bacteria, and animals. Editing DNA can lead to changes in physical traits, like eye colour, and disease risk. Scientists use different technologies to do this." Gene therapies are treatments involving genome editing which aim to prevent and treat diseases in humans. Genome editing tools have the potential to help treat diseases with a genomic basis, like cystic fibrosis and diabetes.

Genome editing is being explored in research on a wide variety of diseases, including single-gene disorders, and it also holds promise for the treatment and prevention of more complex diseases, such as cancer, heart disease, mental illness, and human immunodeficiency virus (HIV) infection.[45]

There is also plenty of research currently into age reversal of our cells by using gene therapy. This is sending a particular piece of DNA to a specific area and having that new DNA implanted into our own. This can either adjust diseased cells or even make the cell younger. This may sound like a far-fetched story, but this has been done by current science and technology in research laboratories. And the effects of making a cell young are likely to be exactly what one would wish for, a rejuvenated body.

---

[45] *What are genome editing and CRISPR-Cas9?: MedlinePlus Genetics.* (n.d.). MedlinePlus.

CRISPR technology

One tool that is now used widely in gene analysis and editing is CRISPR technology. CRISPR enables us to find any gene in the body, like a needle in a haystack. We can also edit the gene with accuracy.

According to an article by The New Scientist, "CRISPR is a technology that can be used to edit genes and, as such, will likely change the world."[46] The article goes on to explain that CRISPR is used to find "a specific bit of DNA inside a cell. After that, the next step in CRISPR gene editing is usually to alter that piece of DNA. However, CRISPR has also been adapted to do other things too, such as turning genes on or off without altering their sequence."

We are already seeing the products of CRISPR technology in other parts of our life, but the potential for it to benefit the healthcare industry should not be underestimated. According to the New Scientist, CRISPR technology has the ability to "transform medicine, enabling us to not only treat but also prevent many diseases."

Science has raced ahead with the possibilities of gene therapy to treat cancers and other diseases.

Car-T treatment

In 2017, the first CAR-T treatment was approved to treat cancer.[47] This treatment uses gene therapy to target our own immune cells and tell them to fight cancer cells. The treatment lets our immune system know exactly what type of cancer is present, rather than just a general message. Our immune system includes T-cells, which are the white blood cells in the body that are primarily responsible for destroying cancerous cells found in tumours. However, they are not always able to recognize the cancer cells. By removing and altering these cells in a lab, they can start to identify the cancer cells better. This makes them more effective in destroying cancerous cells.

---

[46] *What is CRISPR?* (n.d.). New Scientist.
[47] Butera, S. (2018, April 23). *CAR-T: trailblazing the path from clinical development to the clinic*. Gene Therapy.

The treatment has taken decades to develop given its complexity and maintaining the goal of making it as safe as possible. The treatment needs to be completely tailored and personalised to each patient, which is only possible due to many technological advances coming together. For example, even dramatic supply chain advances have been required to ensure that the correct treatment is delivered to the correct patient. The future of this may in fact make medicine simpler, with more ready-made products that we know work well for certain types of people. The cost and availability should then be far better.

Identifying cancer

Cancer identification is becoming much more advanced, with companies now able to analyse the mutated, fractionated DNA and RNA from cancer cells in your blood.

According to Peter Diamandis, "Perhaps the most impactful potential of low-cost genome sequencing is its ability to be used in what is called a liquid biopsy—the ability to find free-flowing cancer DNA in your bloodstream that might indicate the existence of an undetected cancer in your body. And, as we know, finding cancer at stage-zero or stage-one is the key to survival."[48]

As reported in Fierce Biotech, since its 2016 launch, cancer blood test maker Grail has grown to 436 employees and raised nearly $2 billion in venture capital money, including from Bill Gates, Jeff Bezos and many others. That funding has supported a clinical program spanning 115,000 participants, including people with and without cancer, as the company worked to build an atlas of the small, belying pieces of genetic material shed by tumours into the bloodstream.

Earlier this year, Grail demonstrated how its technology could detect more than 50 different types of cancer with a single blood draw while identifying the tumour's tissue of origin 93% of the time.[49]

---

[48] Diamandis, P. H. (n.d.). *100 years old will be the new 60*. Diamandis.
[49] Hale, C. (2020, September 21). *Illumina to pay $8B to reacquire cancer blood test maker Grail, with all eyes on 2021*. FierceBiotech.

Sirtuin genes and spatial transcriptomics

Until recently, it wasn't possible to know how many genes work together or even what their position might be in a single cell. The next generation of scientific understanding can be more precise about gene positions and the interconnectivity of their resultant effects. This is called spatial transcriptomics, which combines precision and breadth to map the work of thousands of genes in individual cells at pinpoint locations in tissue.

Traditional transcriptomics reviews how messenger RNA has effects between genes, but this new level of understanding brings insights into how diseases behave at the gene level. For example, the WCM Weill Cornell Medicine group and others have done spatial analyses of gene activity for other parts of the COVID-19–ravaged body. This new technique can see how cells in the lungs are behaving in a COVID-19 patient, as well as pinpointing how cells in our noses stop functioning and we lose our taste and smell. More importantly, by analysing gene expression in the heart muscle, scientists have found that cells affected by COVID-19 do not function as well as they should even if they look normal from the outside. According to one of the researchers, "Under the microscope the [patients] appear to have a normal number of muscle cells, but if you look at gene expression, it seems the cells have forgotten what they are supposed to be doing."[50] As worrying as this is, it demonstrates how quickly these new technologies are becoming important in our understanding of diseases. It's likely that we are at the beginning of another wave of discoveries of gene expression.

There are some very important research labs across the world researching gene expression of the sirtuin class of genes, in particular, there is the Paul F. Glenn Center for the Biological Mechanisms of Ageing at the Harvard Medical School, where Professor David Sinclair is a co-Director.

The sirtuin genes are the control systems for a wide range of fundamental and critical processes within our bodies. The sirtuin

---

[50] Pennisi, E. (2021, March 18). 'Total game changer': Pinpointing gene activity in tissues is aiding. Science | AAAS.

genes govern the way our body digests food, how the body generates energy, how to heal itself and they help memory function amongst many other critical body functions. Typically, the sirtuin genes are activated in times of difficulty, and the sirtuin genes can put our body into a survival mode, initiating quite magical cellular repair pathways that have existed in organisms from the dawn of life.

There are seven sirtuin genes in humans and each controls different sets of processes. For example, Sirtuin 6 is responsible for regulating DNA repair and telomere maintenance amongst other actions. The importance of these sirtuin genes is really very promising and could the subject of many books. This epigenetic control system of sirtuin genes may indeed hold the promise for far longer lives.

Many of the topics that we are addressing in this book do activate and support the healthy functioning of sirtuin genes, which is why many of the good habits work, such as good sleep, lower calorific intake, and exercise. In the coming chapter, we will look at fasting, intermittent fasting, and positive stress from exercise along with other factors, which help to activate our sirtuin genes and support their functions. In chapter 8 we will go through the various supplements that can also support the sirtuin gene function, thereby giving us an overview of the current research that is addressing ageing medicine.

Future healthcare developments

The creativity with which medicine is able to develop is wonderful. As well as the developments we've already discussed, there is increasing focus on things like the use of exosomes – cellular couriers that shuttle between cells carrying proteins and genetic information – for potentially delivering medication to certain parts of our bodies.[51]

Then there's the creation of virus markers from within our own muscles that can be used within vaccination programmes. One such

---

[51] Cross, R. (2018, July 30). *Meet the exosome, the rising star in drug delivery.* Chemical & Engineering News.

creation is the Imperial College COVID-19 vaccine. According to the Imperial College, "Traditional vaccines are often based on a weakened form of a virus or parts of it, but the Imperial [College] vaccine is based on a new method. Instead, it uses bits of genetic code (called self-amplifying RNA), rather than bits of the virus. Once injected into muscle, the [muscle] cells should produce copies of a protein found on the outside of the virus. This trains the immune system to respond to the coronavirus so the body can easily recognise it as a threat in future."[52]

The above notes on exosomes and self-amplifying RNA are only a spotlight on recent research activity, but I am confident that the future will show incredibly diverse and more exotic healthcare innovations. There are thousands of brilliant people working on longevity science, and we will all benefit from their knowledge as and when it is shared.

---

[52] *How the vaccine works*. (n.d.). Imperial College London

CHAPTER 7:
HOW CAN DIET AND EXERCISE HELP US TO PROLONG OUR LIFESPAN?

As we discussed in earlier chapters, diet is an important factor in maintaining our health and potentially lengthening our lifespan. We've already touched on the diets of those Blue Zone communities and the key components of their food and beverage consumption, and we've looked at how diet can support the health of our telomeres which can support us in the quest for living a longer life. We're now going to take a deeper dive into the different aspects of diets that exist and are, perhaps, popular now, how they fare in the context of increasing our longevity, and some of the additional diet and supplementary options available to us.

Fasting and intermittent fasting

Starting with less diet or missing part of your daily diet. David Sinclair, an expert in longevity science and research, reiterates key findings in science that managing our diet or reducing the calorie intake is the main practical action we can take to support our body toward a longer life. As he wrote in his book, '*Lifespan, Why we age and why we don't have to*', "Your body should be a bellwether and your doctor should let you know if fasting is fine. But if you are in good health, I really couldn't recommend anything better for long-term health than being hungry a little bit during the day". This seems to be quite surprising to me. I've always believed that enough food would keep you healthy, any less would cause problems. But the key thing to realise here, is that David Sinclair is talking about switching on those sirtuin genes that can trigger cellular repair and in effect slow and reverse ageing. The skipping of breakfast so that your body doesn't have food since the evening meal on the day before until lunch the next day is one way to trigger your body to look at rejuvenating energy creation and repair. However, you'll have to eat more at lunch to get to your calorie requirements. It seems important to me to intermittent fast rarely, and never fast if your doctor tells you to eat more regularly. It seems like a very difficult task personally, so I listen to my body and try to eat when it feels right. Sometimes skipping a breakfast just seems to be impossible.

If you're interested in the specific way that Sinclair describes this, "Fasting can activate our survival circuit. The survival circuit is a system that has been in our cells for a long time. It's in all life on the planet. And it serves to keep us alive for longer, healthier for longer, when we're under threat."

He advocates for depriving your body of resources to help it to respond more effectively to survival situations, maintaining the body's ability to stay on form. He concludes: "So when we are doing a bit of exercise, if you run out of breath on the treadmill, that's good. If you're hungry; you skip breakfast and have a late lunch, that's good. This will activate the survival circuit".[53]

Eating to live longer

According to the recently released book *The Telomere Effect: A Revolutionary approach to living younger, healthier, longer*, by health psychologist Elissa Epel and Nobel Prize-winning molecular biologist Elizabeth Blackburn, the whole-food diet is related to longer telomeres, while the diet with large quantities of meat and processed foods is related to shorter telomeres.

They cite oxidative stress (when there are too many free radicals and too few antioxidants) as a key culprit in the shortening of telomeres, and they believe we need antioxidants to neutralise these free radicals. By including lots of antioxidants we keep our level of total oxidative stress low.[54]

[53] Sinclair, D., & LaPlante, M. D. (2019). *Lifespan: Why We Age—and Why We Don't Have To*

[54] Blackburn, E., & Epel, E. (2018). *The Telomere Effect: A Revolutionary Approach to Living Younger, Healthier, Longer*

Our main source of antioxidants is the food we eat – mainly fruits, vegetables and whole grains, which help to maintain strong immune defences and keep our oxidative stress in balance.

Epel and Blackburn suggest the following tips to increase our intake of beneficial antioxidants while eschewing foods that work against us in terms of helpful nutrition.

1) **Choose produce in a rainbow of colours.** Colours reflect the different flavonoids and carotenoids within fruit and vegetables, all of which reduce oxidative stress and inflammation. "Try to include at various times citrus, berries, apples, plums, carrots, green leafy vegetables, tomatoes. There are also antioxidants in beans, nuts, seeds, whole grains, and green tea."

2) **Go for foods rich in omega-3 free fatty acids.** Good choices include certain types of fish, algae (such as seaweed), and walnuts. These help to reduce oxidative stress and inflammation. They advise limiting omega-6 oils such as linoleic acid, found in corn, safflower, sunflower oils and fast food.

3) **Go sparingly on processed meat, processed food, and sugared drinks** Processed meat, for example, is on the World Health Organisation's "probably carcinogenic" list now. Even small reductions in how much processed meat you eat can make a big difference in your health, and the impact on our environment. [55]

Antioxidants are substances that can prevent or slow down any damage to cells that could be caused by free radicals and unstable molecules that the body produces as a reaction to environmental and other pressures.[56]

Glutathione is a powerful antioxidant that is made in our body's cells. Its levels decrease as a result of ageing, stress and exposure to toxins. Boosting glutathione either through our diet or by taking supplements may provide many health benefits. Not surprisingly,

[55] Epel, E. (2017, February 13). *How to Create the Ideal Diet for Telomere Heath*. ELLE.
[56] Ware, M. R. (2018, May 29). *How can antioxidants benefit our health?* Medical News Today.

eating healthy foods supports the production of this antioxidant. Such foods include eggs, grains and vegetables such as onions, mushrooms and broccoli. Regular exercise also correlates to better levels of glutathione in older people. Exercise is not necessarily a cause of those better levels, but the result most likely a correlation with the lifestyle.

Unlike most antioxidants, which come from plant sources, the human body naturally produces glutathione in the liver. However, as we've already said, glutathione levels naturally decrease with age. In fact, researchers found links between low glutathione levels and some age-related conditions, such as glaucoma and macular degeneration (a common condition that affects the middle part of our vision).

In another study, researchers found that whey protein alleviated oxidative stress in human colon cancer cells, which they believed was possible because the protein increased glutathione levels. It has also been found that whey protein can decrease oxidative stress in the lungs of people with cystic fibrosis by increasing glutathione levels.[57]

The importance of fibre

Fibre has long been hailed as an essential food type for maintaining our digestive health, helping us to feel full for longer and fuelling healthy gut bacteria. Fibre is also said to lower cholesterol and blood sugar levels, as well as the risk of cardiovascular diseases and diabetes. Numerous investigations indicate that dietary fibre reduces the risk of disease and premature death. Some of the health benefits associated with dietary fibre could be a result of the preservation of telomeres.[58]

Fibrous foods, particularly plants, contain a substance called 'inulin'. The fibre in inulin is soluble. It dissolves in the stomach and then

[57] Eske, J. (2019, August 30). *4 natural ways to increase glutathione*. Medical News Today.
[58] Tucker, L. A. (2018, April 1). *Dietary Fiber and Telomere Length in 5674 U.S. Adults: An NHANES Study of Biological Ageing*. PubMed Central

forms a gelatinous substance that slows digestion, increases the feeling of fullness and reduces cholesterol absorption as it passes through the digestive tract. Good examples of inulin-rich foods are chicory root, artichokes, agave, asparagus, bananas, garlic, leeks, wheat and onions.[59]

So far, there have been very few investigations focusing on the effect of fibre consumption on biological ageing. Results from a 2018 Nurses' Health Study, indicated that among a variety of dietary factors, fibre intake was directly related to telomere length. A 2017 review by Rafie et al., of a number of other studies examined the relationship between various foods, food groups, and eating patterns and telomere length. Results were mixed. Some of the foods and food groups were shown to be good sources of fibre, such as whole grains, cereals, nuts, legumes, fruits, and vegetables. However, fibre intake was rarely associated with biological ageing.[60]

Most people have gut microbes that are good for us and those gut microbes like inulin fibre. However, other people may have different microbiome gut microbes that could find inulin-rich foods difficult to digest, so it matters who you are and what your gut constitution is. Of course, there are now tests available that can tell you more about your gut health and whether or not your microbiome is sensitive to particular foods or not.

Ketogenic diets and ageing?

We are seeing a rising trend in promotions for ketogenic diets in the press and media. Does a ketogenic diet make your body age or keep you youthful? Probably neither dramatically, but there is analysis of our microbiome by leading dietary companies to suggest that a ketogenic diet *causes ageing* of our digestive system. Fasting or ketogenic diets can produce antioxidants and therefore reduce inflammation; so this is helpful for our bodies. The ketogenic diet also reduces our appetite and causes lower blood sugar levels, both

[59] Watson, K. (2020, March 26). *Benefits of Inulin*. Healthline.
[60] Tucker, L. A. (2018b, April 1). *Dietary Fiber and Telomere Length in 5674 U.S. Adults: An NHANES Study of Biological Ageing*. PubMed Central

likely to bring about behaviour changes that might trigger sirtuin gene activity. However, analysing our microbiome can show increased ageing due to ketogenic diets so on a holistic level ketogenic diets should be approached with some degree of caution over the long term, particularly because this diet isn't balanced across food groups. Negative micro factors could become an issue after a while if you decide to do the ketogenic diet plan.

For those that are curious, similar ageing analysis on our microbiome have determined that a Vegan diet makes your body biological age younger, so that is potentially a more promising longevity diet.

There are many clinics now using ketogenic diets for use in healthcare practice. A patient that is obese, or suffering from early cancer development, or neurological diseases could be suggested to try a ketogenic diet. The diet increases the ketosis of our bodies, which forces the body to burn fats rather than carbohydrates or sugars. Ketosis is a prominent feature of diabetes, so not something to be taken lightly given a ketogenic diet alters our hormones and insulin management. Although some studies are now showing that ketogenic diets can show promising longevity effects in mice, it seems that there are also other signs of trouble for a long-term use of the ketogenic diet; studies are finding increased cholesterol and inflammation.[61] This is obviously quite a powerful diet that can affect our bodies, and so it is an area of much interest before we can draw any conclusions.

The role of nitric oxide in our diets

Nitric oxide is a compound in our body that causes blood vessels to widen and stimulates the release of certain hormones, such as insulin and human growth hormone. It is linked to healthy telomere length and can be generated by using breathing techniques and from consuming certain types of food. Breathing techniques make the most of the nitric oxide that is produced in our nasal cavity. Given

---

[61] Blagosklonny, M.V. (2019) *Fasting and rapamycin: diabetes versus benevolent glucose intolerance.* Cell Death & Disease

that these techniques are free to try, it should be your first port of call to boost healthy nitric oxide levels.

There are nitric oxide supplements available too that doctors sometimes prescribe. The two most common nitric oxide supplements are L-arginine and L-citrulline. But each of these supplements is found naturally in our common fresh foods. L-arginine is an amino acid, a protein building block, which is usually found in red meat, dairy products, poultry, and fish. L-citrulline is also an amino acid found naturally in meat, nuts, legumes and fruits such as watermelon.

Many people think that increasing nitric oxide in our bodies will enhance blood flow in the body to improve performance in sports, promote healing, enhance heart health, and provide many other potential benefits.[62]

Can exercise impact our age?

Experts generally agree that keeping active is essential for good health and can also impact the length of our telomeres. A study published in November 2018 in the *European Heart Journal* compared different types of training on telomere length and telomerase activity.

The study involved 124 people over a six month period. Participants were split into four groups, with each group focused on either endurance training, high-intensity interval training (HIIT), resistance training, or one control group.
Each exercise group was instructed to do three 45-minute sessions of their assigned type of training each week. The telomere length and telomerase activity were measured in the participants' white blood cells before and after the study.

According to the lead researcher of the study, Ulrich Laufs, the main finding was that, "Compared to the start of the study and the control

---

[62] Nall, R. M. (2019, September 19). *What to know about nitric oxide supplements*. Medical News Today.

group, in volunteers who did endurance and high-intensity training, the telomerase activity and telomere length increased, which are both important for cellular ageing, regenerative capacity and thus, healthy ageing. Interestingly, resistance training did not exert these effects."

So, endurance training (cardio) and HIIT were shown to positively impact telomere health by working to lengthen telomeres, but resistance training had no effect.[63] That is not to say there is no health benefit to practising resistance training. Weight training continues to be important in maintaining our strength in muscle tissue and bone as we age. Bone density becomes an issue as we get older because it can increase our frailty and likelihood of accidents. Strength training can increase bone density and thereby hopefully boost our resilience to life's knocks and bumps.

There is growing consensus that for every hour you are exercising, you're adding a large multiple of that to your life. So for example, if you are doing five workouts of thirty minutes a week, then this would be two and a half hours a week, which would be multiplied by around seven times resulting in seventeen and a half extra hours being added to your life for every week of exercise. Over time, this would add up, so that a years' worth of that exercise regime would an extra thirty eight days of healthy life. Stick to that exercise for over thirty years, and you'll accumulate three years and one and a half months of extra life. Those extra years are perhaps time you wouldn't have had at all, and most likely a later stage of life without exercise would be diseased, miserable and suffer from expensive medical care. This illustration is just a general musing, but one that is likely to hold true if further research backs up initial findings.

Bespoke diets

There are many highly popular (and famous) diets available for people to follow these days, such as the Mediterranean diet, paleo,

[63] Moore, R. (2021, January 2). *Is It Possible to Lengthen Telomeres With Diet & Exercise?* Visual Impact Fitness.

ketogenic, Atkins, vegetarian and vegan. Weight loss is often, but not always, the main objective or rationale behind choosing one of these types of diets. Some of them may be prescribed by health professionals to achieve certain health goals; some may be chosen for other considerations such as climate change or animal welfare. The reasons for sticking to a particular diet may be less diverse. Most often, someone drops a diet because the goal has been achieved (weight loss or health correction), or it is too complex to fit into their lifestyle. The simple fact is, no one 'type' of diet is perfect for every single person because we each have a gut microbiome as unique as our fingerprint.[64] It is our gut microbiomes that dictate our personal diet requirements. For this reason, possibly the best diet you can find and thrive on is one that is tailored to be bespoke to you.

Some people may not benefit from certain healthy foods, and the more we know about the details of our microbiome gut health, the better we can prescribe nutrients to support us and increase our lifespan. This will potentially be a part of our regular monitoring in the future, and it is already possible today.

In summary, nutrition is clearly an essential factor in our ageing and longevity but is a complex matter with so many different diets, food types and supplements available to impact the various parts and functions of our body. Some people react differently to healthy foods and nutrients, and so no one answer for a perfect diet will work. This is where I think artificial intelligence will help us to make great strides forward in this area. The most amazing thing about artificial intelligence is that it's transforming scientific knowledge about diet and bringing answers to our table. We are beginning to understand the most complicated systems in our bodies more than ever, and can use nutrition to help fight cancers, diabetes, cardiovascular diseases and many more before they even get started.

---

[64] *What Diet is Best for Me? Paleo? Keto? Vegan?* (2018, June 29). Viome.

CHAPTER 8:

SERIOUSLY POWERFUL SUPPLEMENTS. ARE LONGEVITY DAILY DOSES OF METFORMIN, RAPAMYCIN AND NAD+ BOOSTER NMN WORTH CONSIDERING?

As we discussed in the previous chapter, the ability we now have to know exactly what our bodies like, don't like, need and will benefit from, is unprecedented. So, too, is the range of options available to us in the world of supplementation and preventative medicine. Here, I'm going to discuss a few more options that have been found to have some impact towards the extension of lifespan: Metformin, Rapamycin and Nicotinamide Mononucleotide (NMN) amongst others. Scientific researchers are working hard to understand the detail of where and when these will work best. If it's not these miracle substances that extend our healthy lifespan, we will find other and more promising options. I also want to say that the discovery of each of these is simply miraculous for medicine in general. The results from these drugs have helped millions of people with specific diseases. And going forward, it is so exciting to see what else the discoveries will be used for to help with disease and healthy ageing.

NAD+ booster nicotinamide mononucleotide (NMN)

This relatively recent trend of taking supplements to support cell mechanics is being further supported by the leading research by David Sinclair, and he summarises this in the book, *Lifespan, Why We Age and Why We Don't Have To.* The science behind these supplements is still being investigated, but some people are starting to see benefits by experimenting on themselves. This is a fairly high-risk strategy, where you could reduce your lifespan, or give yourself a disease, all while trying to live longer and more healthily.

Nicotinamide Adenine Dinucleotide (NAD+) is the most abundant molecule in our bodies after water. It is essential for life and energy processes in our cells. NAD+ is used in the transfer of electrons in and around our cells, and so is vital for all of our cellular processes.

As we discussed earlier in this book, one aspect of ageing is a decrease in DNA repair as well as effective energy production in cells. DNA repairing mechanisms require NAD+, which supports the repairing sirtuin genes' actions. We know that NAD+ declines with ageing, so people are now experimenting with taking supplements to boost NAD+ to support the DNA repairing process. These supplements include Nicotinamide Mononucleotide (NMN), which increases our body's production of NAD+.

Amongst other compounds, Sinclair is focusing on NMN, which is a molecule that naturally occurs in all living things are comes from B vitamins in our body. NMN is then turned into NAD+. It's practical for NMN to be the supplement instead of NAD+ because it's difficult for our bodies to absorb the latter larger molecule, whereas the NMN is more readily absorbed. Sinclair is keen to research NMN given it is considered safe and non-toxic and hasn't been shown to have side effects yet. So if this supplement is tested rigorously then we may have found a useful ingredient to result in DNA repair.

NAD+ has been a subject of research for many decades for its abundance in the body and its crucial role in keeping our bodies running. In non-human studies, raising NAD+ levels in the body have shown promising results in age-related disease, and has also shown some anti-ageing properties.

Some studies suggest it can be used to positively impact age-related illnesses such as diabetes, cardiovascular diseases, neurodegeneration and general decreases in the immune system.

Its effects on heart function have also been explored, to an extent, and studies have shown that boosting NAD+ levels can protect the heart and improve cardiac functions, albeit in mice.

In a separate study using mice with Alzheimer's, raising the NAD+ level showed a decrease in the protein build-up that disrupts cell communication in the brain, presenting a new possible approach to tackling neurodegeneration.

And further studies have suggested that NAD+ levels play an important role in regulating inflammation and cell survival during the immune response and ageing.[65]

This all leads to NMN being a very exciting supplement with huge promise in research. It fits all of the necessary requirements so far for a component to support longevity.

Metformin

One promising drug treatment that is gaining a large following from people seeking a longer lifespan is metformin. It is the drug most commonly used in the management of diabetes, and one that diabetics have been prescribed for many years. The medicine works in diabetics by lowering the amount of sugar the body produces and absorbs. As it lowers glucose production in the liver, metformin also lowers blood sugar by increasing the body's sensitivity to insulin. It also decreases the amount of glucose that our bodies absorb from the foods we eat.[66] The dosage needs to be carefully prescribed, so a doctor or physician determines how much a patient should have.

In research into the effects of metformin, evidence from animal models and in vitro studies suggest that in addition to its effects on glucose metabolism, metformin may influence metabolic and cellular processes associated with the development of age-related conditions. So it seems from much research that metformin can

---

[65] *What is NMN?* (2021, May 11). NMN.com.
[66] *Everything You Always Wanted to Know About Metformin, But Were Afraid to Ask.* (2021, March 18). DiaTribe.

reduce inflammation, lower oxidative damage, improve autophagy, and reduce cell senescence.[67]

While giving metformin to healthy people *might* help delay ageing, doctors are reluctant to prescribe it for that specific purpose without official guidance. Doctors can prescribe metformin off-label, but people must assess the risks themselves. "Off-label" use means that the medicine is being used in a way that is different to that which is described in the drug licence.

Metformin is one of many drugs that are called mTOR protein inhibitors. These drugs get in the way of the natural cell division in our bodies (mTOR drives our body's growth). By turning the mTOR protein activity down, researchers believe the drug can also provide similar benefits to those seen as a result of calorie-restrictive diets and intermittent fasting. The way that metformin works will really depend upon the diet that we have.[68] As nutrition is complicated, it will be very important for scientists to do plenty of research on how metformin impacts our bodies and what effects are compounded by diet changes.

Some ambitious researchers have designed scientific trials that would interrogate the possibility of metformin positively impacting lifespan, but they struggle to obtain financing. These scientists want to specifically see if metformin delays or averts cancers, dementia, stroke and heart attacks, but we won't know for a long time if metformin will be a proven drug for these purposes.

Rapamycin

Rapamycin (also known as Sirolimus or Rapamune or Everolimus) is a low-cost, fairly generic drug that is used to help suppress people's immune systems after they've received an organ transplant. It also

---

[67] *Metformin in Longevity Study (MILES). - Full Text View - ClinicalTrials.gov.* (n.d.). Clinical Trials.

[68] Palliyaguru, D. L., Minor, R. K., Mitchell, S. J., Palacios, H. H., Licata, J. J., Ward, T. M., Abulwerdi, G., Elliott, P., Westphal, C., Ellis, J. L., Sinclair, D. A., Price, N. L., Bernier, M., & de Cabo, R. (2020). *Combining a High Dose of Metformin With the SIRT1 Activator, SRT1720, Reduces Life Span in Aged Mice Fed a High-Fat Diet.* The Journals of Gerontology: Series A

has been shown to suppress senescent cells, which we have already discussed would help reduce age-related diseases. And this is reason enough for some people to start self-experimenting with the drug, with the aim of increasing their lifespan. It has reportedly been found to lengthen the lives of old mice by 9 to 14 per cent and boost longevity in flies and yeast.

Rapamycin has been found to strongly suppress the immune system, which is why it is often given to people who receive new organs, to stop them from rejecting their transplants.

Rapamycin blocks a protein called TOR ("target of rapamycin"), the first known protein that influences longevity in the four species that scientists commonly use to study ageing: yeast, worms, flies and mice.

A recent article in the publication *Nature* suggests it might be worth further research, as the longevity benefits seem to be found across different studies, and side effects are minor, so long as the dosage is correct.[69]

To me, it seems like the jury is still out on rapamycin drug usage for the general public. It holds vast promise for longevity and could be a wonder drug in the future. It works similarly to intermittent fasting and very low-calorie diets, which all have the same positive effects on our bodies with improved insulin sensitivity, and most likely some activation of the sirtuin genes and suppression of cellular senescence. We will see how this area develops.

Resveratrol

NAD+, and the supplement NMN in turn, helps another useful compound, Resveratrol, to work effectively. Resveratrol is a compound that various plants create in order to fight off bacteria, fungi and other microbial attackers, or to withstand drought or lack

---

[69] Blagosklonny, M.V. (2019). *Fasting and rapamycin: diabetes versus benevolent glucose intolerance*. Nature.

of nutrients. It has been found in red and purple grapes, blueberries, cranberries, mulberries, lingonberries, peanuts, and pistachios. It is thought to activate the beneficial sirtuin genes and therefore promote the associated cellular pathways to reduce inflammation and promote repair.

Virtually all of the positive studies on Resveratrol have been performed using cultures of cells, or lab tests with yeast, worms, flies and mice. The few human studies have looked at specific intermediate markers, such as levels of antioxidants, heart rate variability, blood flow to the brain, and amounts of cancer proteins. None have measured long-term health in humans or survival yet.

Another big unknown relating to Resveratrol is the side effects of taking it as a supplement. Resveratrol, despite being difficult for our bodies to absorb, acts on many different tissues in the body. It is chemically related to the hormone oestrogen and in some situations, high doses of Resveratrol boost the activity of oestrogen, while in others it blocks oestrogen. That would make Resveratrol supplements somewhat risky for women who have a history of suffering from cancer of the breast, ovary, uterus, or other oestrogen-sensitive tissue; those trying to become pregnant; or those taking an oral contraceptive.[70]

Coenzyme Q10

There are almost endless supplements that could be interesting. And one potentially lesser-known supplement is starting to become more researched for lifespan enhancement. Coenzyme Q10 is an important vitamin-like substance that is known to be required for the proper function of many organs and chemical reactions in the body. It helps to provide energy to our cells because it helps our mitochondria to function. Coenzyme Q10 also seems to promote antioxidant activity, thereby reducing inflammation in our cells.

People with certain diseases such as heart failure, high blood pressure, gum disease, Parkinson's disease, blood infections, certain

---

[70] Harvard Health. (2012, February 3). *Resveratrol—the hype continues.*

diseases of the muscles and HIV infection, might have lower levels of coenzyme Q10 and as a result, are sometimes prescribed this as a supplement. There are now people taking Q10 as a preventative supplement to support their cells' functions and stave off future diseases related to ageing. Experts are yet to determine the longer-term benefits.

Phosphatidylcholine

Another supplement that is becoming more popular is Phosphatidylcholine. Abbreviated to PC, this supplement is traditionally used to support brain health, it can also support liver function and keep cholesterol levels in check.[71]

PC can be obtained naturally through the diet, in foods such as eggs, broccoli, mustard, soy beans or sunflower (seeds or oil). It is thought to be possible that PC can positively impact many health issues because it improves a common causative factor behind them - the integrity and health of your cell membranes. The PC level in your body is an essential factor in maintaining, or improving, the robustness of your cell membranes. And it is found in good supply in centenarians.

Benefits of taking PC are said to include:
1) Improved memory performance and learning during the ageing process
2) Reduction of inflammation in stress conditions
3) Reduction of cholesterol and triglyceride levels
4) Reduction of fat deposits
5) Alleviation of PMS and painful menstruation
6) Reduction of medication side effects
7) Improved exercise performance[72]

---

[71] McDermott, A. (2018, September 18). *What Is Phosphatidylcholine and How Is It Used?* Healthline.
[72] Garma, J. (2019, July 19). *7 Phosphatidylcholine Benefits That Can Improve Your Long-term Health*. ProHealth Longevity.

PC is also used for treating hepatitis, eczema, gallbladder disease and circulation problems.[73] Perfect, fingers crossed right? As you may have come to guess, I will of course suggest that further studies in this area are likely to yield some actionable results, and so we hope that research will uncover breakthrough science with how Phosphatidylcholine may help support our body and reduce diseases.

In summary

The purpose of this chapter is to give you a sense of what supplements are currently being explored. Progress is being made to positively impact ageing. The supplements I've mentioned in this chapter also highlight that the scientific community is still at an early stage in being able to draw solid conclusions about safety and effectiveness.

My takeaway from this chapter is that I would prefer to wait until the scientific community is able to make more solid, proven statements about the benefits and possible side effects of these supplements. Some seem like they would have very severe consequences is if the dosage is incorrect, so I worry about people taking Metformin, Rapamycin and Resveratrol for example. Getting a dose correct may sound easy, but I think people need lots of help and additional guidance from their doctor or physician to ensure supplements are not damaging. We may also realise that given each of us is unique, the supplements may not work exactly as intended, leading to more bespoke advice. There is still a long way to go but it is reassuring to know that the appetite to dig deeper is there and I look forward to future findings and developments in this fascinating field of study.

---

[73] *Phosphatidylcholine: Health Benefits, Uses, Side Effects, Dosage & Interactions.* (2019, September 17). RxList.

CHAPTER 9:
STEM CELL REPLENISHMENT, THE NEXT FRONTIER

Despite thousands of clinics and businesses offering stem cell replenishment, it is still a controversial topic. Mostly because, at this stage, the general use of stem cells is unproven and unlicensed, and yet there are a very large number of services facilitating this, available to the general public. It is hoped that regulations will be tightened to ensure broader safety.[74]

What is stem cell therapy?

Stem-cell therapy is the use of stem cells to treat or prevent a disease or condition. It refers to the extraction of stem cells from certain parts of the body, which are then used in treatments for neurodegenerative diseases and conditions such as diabetes and heart disease.

Stem cell therapy is interesting because there may be more benefits to the use of this type of therapy in addressing spinal cord injuries, type 1 diabetes, Parkinson's disease, heart disease, and osteoarthritis amongst others.

The extracted cells can change to become any other type of cell that is required in our body to function such as blood cells, brain cells, heart muscle cells or bone cells.[75]

---

[74] Wikipedia contributors. (2021, May 6). *Stem-cell therapy*. Wikipedia.
[75] NHS website. (2020, May 5). *Stem cell and bone marrow transplants*. NHS. UK.

As well as the ability to 'differentiate' into another cell type with a specialised function, stem cells are also characterised by the fact that they can divide and multiply to form copies of themselves. These two distinct properties mean stem cells can serve as an internal repair system, dividing without limit to replenish other cells.[76]

The way it works is, researchers grow stem cells in a lab, which they have either taken from the patient's own body or possibly a donor. Those researchers then manipulate the cells to become specific types of cells and those cells are then transferred to the patient. Researchers have already shown that adult stem cells derived from bone marrow, which are guided to become heart-like cells, can repair heart tissue in patients. Such findings have triggered a great deal of interest within the medical and scientific communities, so further research is being undertaken as we speak.

Scientists have even managed to take normal adult cells (not stem cells) and reprogram them to go back to an embryonic stem cell state, and then grow into other useful cells for our bodies. I believe that this area of development is going to be life-changing. Having access to this type of therapy will hel26p to boost our bodies' ability to repair itself in ways that would seem miraculous nowadays.

The positive outcomes of stem cell therapy are bountiful. Some results have shown that stem cells can boost a patient's immune system to fight some types of cancer and blood-related diseases, such as leukaemia and lymphoma.

There is some controversy surrounding stem-cell therapy following developments such as the ability of scientists to isolate and culture embryonic stem cells, to create stem cells using somatic cell nuclear transfer (a strategy for creating a viable embryo from a body cell and an egg cell), and their use of techniques to create induced pluripotent stem cells (considered to be 'master' cells). This controversy is often related to viewpoints on abortion and human cloning.

---

[76] *Stem cell (cell replacement) therapy.* (n.d.). European Parkinson's Disease Association.

There is also controversy about the source of stem cells in cases where a stem cell donor is used. There are far more stem cells in our bodies when we're young and even before we are born when we are just an embryo. Researchers are using stem cells from embryos for a variety of tests, although this is still rare in research laboratories due to restricted funding and licences.

To me, this is a complex issue, steeped in conflicting viewpoints, and perhaps if this is an important ethical question to you, then this particular therapy may not sound appealing. The Mayo Clinic in the US also highlights that using embryonic stem cells in adults can grow irregularly or specialize in different cell types spontaneously and might also trigger an immune response in which the patient's body thinks the stem cells are foreign invaders and attacks them. There is also the chance that the stem cells might simply fail to function normally, and the consequences of this are as yet, unknown.

Treating Parkinson's disease with stem cell therapy

Sufferers of Parkinson's disease don't have enough dopamine in their bodies. This is a chemical that allows messages to be sent to the parts of the brain that control movement and some forms of thinking. Parkinson's disease kills dopamine-producing nerve cells, or neurons, in some parts of the brain but not others, which may explain why other symptoms exist, such as sleep, motivation and thought.[77]

As dopamine nerve cells die, Parkinson's sufferers develop tremors and rigidity, and their movements, on the whole, slow down. They may also lose their sense of smell or suffer from sleep disorders, depression, constipation, and sometimes dementia in the later stages of the disease, as it spreads out to affect other nerve cells.

Scientists are still confused by what causes Parkinson's. In around one in 20 cases, it is caused by a genetic problem that affects the production of the alpha-synuclein protein. It is unclear what causes the remaining 95 per cent of cases.

---

[77] *Parkinson's disease: how could stem cells help?* (n.d.). Eurostemcell.

The aim of stem cell research in Parkinson's disease is to understand how nerve cells develop, why some of them die, and how healthy cells can be used to replace the damaged brain cells. With this knowledge, researchers are finding that it may be possible to replace the damaged cells in the brain by introducing healthy dopamine-producing cells generated from stem cells that have been grown in the laboratory. Healthy dopamine-producing cells derived from stem cells could also be useful to researchers in testing new treatments for the disease.

Researchers are particularly interested in exploring embryonic stem cells, as they have the potential to develop into all types of cells in the body, including the brain. It is widely acknowledged that more research is needed in order to understand the way these cells work, to ensure that any replication can be controlled, and a safe treatment developed.[78]

Stem cell therapy to reverse ageing

Because Studies have shown that stem cells can regenerate damaged or diseased tissues, reduce inflammation and modulate the immune system, it is perhaps unsurprising that there are now many private clinics that offer stem cell transplants to treat otherwise largely healthy patients who simply want to slow down the ageing process.

As we age, the quantity and function of our stem cells decline, until eventually, the old or damaged cells cannot be replaced, a contributing factor to ageing. The use of regenerative therapies to reverse ageing lies in minimising the gradual decline in stem cell quantity and function, replace them, or boost the function of the remaining ones. For example, there have been studies in mice to replace stem cells in the brain, which have provided evidence of an improvement in the way that the ageing brain can function.[79]

---

[78] *Stem cell (cell replacement) therapy.* (n.d.). European Parkinson's Disease Association.

[79] Evangelou, C. (2020, January 17). *Using stem cells to reverse ageing?* Longevity.Technology.

This field of scientific research is going to become increasingly important as we learn more about how to use stem cell therapy safely, to benefit more people in general, as well as treat severe diseases. The possibility that we can reprogram our DNA, and then use that improved DNA in stem cells that can heal us perfectly, is truly breath-taking. Not only that, but the possibility for stem cells to find weak areas of our body's cells and support them, really brings rejuvenation and regeneration to a whole other level. We could quite literally have a youthful body, youthful cells and greater athleticism ahead in our lifetime. Upending the notion that our best physical days are behind us.

CHAPTER 10:
THERAPY, HEALING THE MIND
FOR THE LONG-TERM

The importance of good mental health

Mental health refers to our emotional, psychological, and social well-being. It affects how we think, feel, and act, and it also helps determine how we handle stressful situations, how we relate to others, and the choices we make about our lifestyle and wellbeing. Mental health is important throughout our whole life as different 'seasons' of life can present different challenges for us.

Mental and physical health are equally important components of overall health. Mental illness, especially depression, increases the risk for many types of physical health problems, particularly long-lasting conditions like the likelihood of having a stroke, type 2 diabetes, and heart disease.

Inversely, the presence of chronic conditions can increase the risk for mental illness. And importantly the effect can be controlled to our advantage. For example, it has been found that our mental health can have an impact on our immune system functions. One study indicated that immune system functions are increased due to psychotherapies such as behaviour therapy, cognitive therapy, or supportive therapy, amongst others. The study, which involved 4,060 participants, found that some of those psychosocial interventions, e.g. cognitive behaviour therapy (CBT), were associated with enhanced immune system function. Overall, being randomly assigned to a psychosocial intervention condition versus a control condition was associated with a 14.7% improvement in beneficial immune system function and an 18.0% decrease in harmful immune system function over time.[80]

Mental health and ageing

The evidence of us ageing is not only viewed as the current status of our health or any diseases we may be suffering from, but how we look, physically. The way we look has been largely attributed to the genes handed down through our parents, the physical exercise we do and what we feed our bodies. What is less likely to be considered is the effect of our mental health on the way we look.

However, research has shown that our mental health affects how others perceive our physical appearance – and whether they want to befriend us. As we discussed earlier in this book, a positive mindset in itself can be a tool in our life-prolonging arsenal. In support of that, we need good mental health, unmuddied by underlying esteem issues or lingering emotional reactions from major life events, for example.

While there are techniques that can help a person to nurture a more positive mindset, a basis of good mental health can often only be achieved with the help of professional therapy. And not only can it form the foundational pillars for a development of a positive mindset and the renewed sense of self that can sometimes be derived from therapy, but it can also impact other aspects of your life and wellbeing, which can ultimately contribute to a longer lifespan. Some of the long-term benefits of therapy may include:

- Helping you to learn life-long coping skills – giving you the tools to manage stressful situations whenever they appear. A therapist can get to know your unique coping strategies and help you to foster these accordingly. Different therapists may teach different strategies for your approach to life. For example, cognitive behavioural therapists (CBT) will also help you to re-train your inner dialogue, so you are less impacted by what others think.

---

[80] Shields, G. S. (2020, October 1). *Psychosocial Interventions and Immune System Function: A Systematic Review and Meta-analysis of Randomized Clinical Trials.* PubMed.

- Changing the way you interact with people – a good therapist can help you become aware of any positive or negative habitual behaviour you display towards others, and help you to understand your boundaries and how you should expect others to treat you
- Making you feel happier – therapy can help you to better understand yourself which then leads to a feeling of compassion towards yourself. Greater compassion will lead you to give yourself more respect, so you won't always find yourself in positions you wished you weren't in because you sold yourself short, for example.
- Leading to improved learning – according to Shawn Achor, author of *The Happiness Advantage*, "Happiness gives us a real chemical edge...How? Positive emotions flood our brains with dopamine and serotonin, chemicals that not only make us feel good, but [also] dial up the learning centres of our brains to higher levels".
- Helping to improve chronic stress – by teaching you methods for calming your mind, identifying what is causing you stress, and techniques to reduce stress without help, you'll greatly lower the longer-term stress of your mind.

In this context, we should think of therapy as a way to improve our mental health, just as we would regard exercise as a way of improving our physical health. According to therapists Anne Floyd and Rob Winkler who outlined the benefits above, "Therapy is not about fixing something that is broken: instead, it is about embracing what we have in order to reach our full, prosperous potential as human beings."[81]

Talking therapies and their benefits

Talking therapy is perhaps the most common type of therapy and is professionally guided talking. Your therapist will likely ask you some questions to encourage you to open up about aspects of your life and childhood, that might give some clues as to how and why you

[81] Hollstadt, N. (2020, November 22). *David Hoy and Associates*. David Hoy & Associates.

may be finding things difficult in your life right now. The therapist isn't there to give you answers or support every decision you make; they are there to help you to evaluate your own thoughts and actions, in a safe, confidential space. Talking through difficult subjects can help your brain to process them better, lessening the damaging effect those subjects might be having on your mental wellbeing. It also helps to feel as though you are being listened to without judgement.

Cognitive Behavioural Therapy (CBT) is also a talk-based therapy, based on the premise that your thoughts, feelings, physical responses and actions are all connected, and that negative thoughts and feelings can trap you in a cycle of negative thinking.

CBT aims to help you deal with overwhelming problems in a more positive way by breaking them down into smaller parts. Your therapist will provide tools and techniques to change negative patterns to improve the way you feel.

Unlike some other talking therapies, CBT deals with your current concerns, rather than focusing on issues from your past. It looks for practical ways to improve your state of mind on a daily basis.[82]

Psychodynamic therapy is another talk-based therapy. According to Good Therapy, a US-based resource for people to find the right type of therapy and the right therapist for their needs, "Psychodynamic therapy is the psychological interpretation of mental and emotional processes. Rooted in traditional psychoanalysis, it draws from object relations, ego psychology, and self-psychology. It was developed as a simpler, less-lengthy alternative to psychoanalysis."

Psychodynamic therapy aims to address the foundation and formation of psychological processes. In this way, it seeks to reduce symptoms and improve people's lives.

---

[82] NHS website. (2021, February 25). *Overview - Cognitive behavioural therapy (CBT)*. NHS. UK.

The therapists help people gain insight into their lives and present-day problems. To do this, together with the patient, they will review certain life factors, including emotions, thoughts, early-life experiences and beliefs. By recognizing recurring patterns the therapist can identify ways in which a person can avoid distress or develop defence mechanisms enabling them to cope better.[83]

Group therapy is another form of talk-based therapy. According to the mental healthcare provider, The Priory Group, there is considerable evidence to show there are clear benefits in treating a range of mental health disorders in a group environment. "Group therapy offers something unique to any other way of delivering treatment - the support, shared experience and thoughts of your peers, as well as those of a professional. You may be struggling with a loss or a trauma for example, and groups can be a support network that provides the opportunity to meet others experiencing similar concerns."

During group therapy sessions, each patient is encouraged to share their experiences and work on understanding themselves in a compassionate and therapeutic environment. Some of the positive outcomes are said to include i) giving people the freedom to express themselves without feeling judged, ii) developing peoples' compassion towards themselves and others, iii) giving patients hope as they see others progress, iv) helping patients to feel safe, and v) encouraging patients to model healthy behaviours and attachments.

We identified that people in the Blue Zones often show signs of communal relationships and group meaning. I believe that group therapy can have a significant effect towards achieving communal and social group meaning. And therefore, group therapy is likely to build those same foundations seen in Blue Zones for people who really need it, to live longer together.

---

[83] Good Therapy Editor Team. (n.d.). *Psychodynamic Therapy*. Good Therapy.

Post-traumatic stress disorder

Therapy to help with trauma and disease in our life is becoming more mainstream. The benefits are being better understood, and health practitioners can bring psychotherapies into the treatment plans to support recovery.

We are even finding that there are ways to cure post-traumatic stress disorder (PTSD) using psychedelic drugs. It's important to remember that PTSD doesn't just affect soldiers and others who work in hazardous professions, but it also affects many of us during significant life events such as giving birth.

Childbirth is widely regarded as being one of the most profound experiences a mother can have, but it is not uncommon for the experience to trigger PTSD. Typical symptoms include flashbacks, nightmares, obsessive thoughts and emotional distress.

A study of 1,500 women showed that if the woman's immediate emotional response to childbirth is particularly negative, it is a very strong indicator that they might eventually develop PTSD in the long term. Researchers are now looking into whether an intervention of the 'feel good' hormone oxytocin in the first days after giving birth could improve maternal bonding and decrease any kind of stress response following the childbirth experience.[84]

Finding a silver lining to every cloud

Having a positive outlook is far more enjoyable than having a negative one if only to relieve the people around you. And there are many more benefits to being a more optimistic thinker. There is research to suggest optimistic people have a reduced risk of heart disease, stroke and lung-related problems. Optimism is also associated with a lower risk of early death from diseases such as cancer, and serious infections. And now a new study links optimism to living a longer life.[85]

---

[84] *What Is Postpartum PTSD?* (2020, May 27). Goop.
[85] Harvard Health. (2019, October 16). *If you are happy and you know it... you may live longer.*

The study outlined in *Proceedings of the National Academy of Sciences* found that people who had higher levels of optimism had a longer lifespan. We noted this in chapter 2, but what are the reasons why optimism affects longevity? While the study wasn't designed to explain this, the researchers shared their views on the matter. While one component of optimism appears to be genetic, the other factor is that our environment and our approach to learning also shape our level of optimism.[86]

So, how can we find ways to give ourselves some helpful therapy on the road to nurture our sense of optimism?

- By reframing situations to see any positive aspects of the situation
- Make time each day to focus on the positive, such as what has made you happy or proud?
- Practice gratitude meditation by taking some time to sit quietly, clear your head on focus on the things you are thankful for
- Spend time with friends and neighbours to make you feel connected, valued and supported
- Set specific and achievable goals each day to grow your confidence in your abilities
- Fake it 'til you make it. Smile as often as you can remind yourself to, as this will help re-train your brain into thinking you are happy.[87]

So we know that loneliness and the associations of despair, depression and anxiety will shorten your life. One of the really fun things to do as we age is to keep up to date with what is happening in the world around us. One of the best ways to keep seeing fresh perspectives is to work with or have friends that are younger than you. Multigenerational living also helps achieve this. It's wonderful to be younger, and spending time with people that help you to live life more fully, and more meaningfully, is probably the most fun part of self-care for longevity, and, potentially, is the whole point of life, anyway.

---

[86] Lee, L. O. (2019, September 10). *Optimism is associated with exceptional longevity in 2 epidemiologic cohorts of men and women*. PubMed.
[87] Harvard Health. (2019b, October 16). *If you are happy and you know it. . . you may live longer*.

CHAPTER 11:

ENERGY AND MAGNETISM

Energy therapies are therapies that involve the use of various types of energy fields on our bodies. According to the US National Center for Complementary and Integrative Health, the goal of energy therapies is to bring energy into the patient or balance the energy within a patient.

Research has shown that energetic and magnetic treatment bands have no extra effect on people who wear them, other than placebo. However, the principles behind energetic and magnetic therapies are worth further consideration in my opinion. While this topic as a whole could be a little more alternative than those we've covered so far, I do believe there is some merit in bringing energetic medicine knowledge into our current picture of healthspan and lifespan. This is not research-driven material but collated insights from a field of alternative medicine that could lead to greater understanding in the future. I recommend you read through this chapter with an open mind, and you might find some ideas interesting.

There are many kinds of energy therapies, some of which use treatments such as light, sound, and magnets. These treatments are relatively easy to measure. Other kinds of energy therapies, such as Healing Touch, Reiki, Qigong and therapeutic touch, which are intended to affect energy fields that surround and penetrate the human body, are potentially not as easy to measure or research.[88] Some of these therapies are incredibly old and learned by people

---

[88] Bach, M. (n.d.). *What Are Energy Therapies?* Taking Charge of Your Health & Wellbeing.

throughout very long and mastered careers, which is not an area I know well.

In medicine, there was something that caught my attention though, and it is to do with the pH or voltage and electricity in our body.

Energetic Medicine

Energetic Medicine has been developed by a doctor in the US called Jerry Tennant. He aimed to discover how the body uses electricity to function. The key learning he found was that each of our cells is designed to run at a specific voltage and a specific frequency. His book describes that "every cell in the body is designed to run at -20 to -25 millivolts. To heal, we must make new cells. To make a new cell requires -50 millivolts." Interestingly enough, he also noticed that disease correlates to when cells have too little voltage and are running at too low a frequency.

Dr Tennant summarised that the main aspects that control voltage are the thyroid hormone, fulvic acid, dental infections, scars and exercise amongst others.

Amongst some advice, he advises good dental hygiene and dental operations to maintain healthy energy pathways. There are also plenty of homeopathic and diet tips to consider in his book, *Healing Voltage*, mostly focusing on eating unprocessed food and drinking plenty of clean water.

The nutrition we have in our lives should supply the right pH levels, or, let's say, the right voltage. Water can be healthier if it is alkaline. Fluids such as alcohol and coffee are less healthy for our bodies because they are not alkaline; the voltage is disrupted by alcohol, for example, and our cells function less well in Dr Tennant's opinion.

The Tennant Institute's Health Protocol is based on the belief that if your body can consistently regenerate good cells, then it can heal itself.

The muscles in our body are able to act as battery storage for the voltage that is required in our cells. By taking a walk, or doing exercise, we boost the voltage in our muscles, which can then energise the cells surrounding it. The muscle fascia that wraps the outside can act as pathways to distribute the energy. Also, each organ will have some version of its own battery using smaller layers of muscles. These muscle groups and layers may be more commonly known to you as Meridian lines developed from ancient Chinese medicine. This now may all start to make sense to you as there are different areas of science and medicine that describe the same health and repair mechanisms. Science will incorporate all of these aspects over time, but for now, these areas lay outside the realm of US-based physicians.[89]

Magnetic therapy

Magnetic therapy is another form of energetic healing. It is an ancient practice, reportedly dating back at least 2,000 years. It most commonly uses the power of static magnets to achieve numerous health benefits.

The concept is based on the fact that iron makes up around four per cent of our blood content, and every ion in our cells carries an electrical charge. This makes up our bodies own electrical field, which means that when the negative side of the magnet is placed on a painful area of our body, it draws fresh oxygenated blood to that area. It is thought that magnetic therapy can improve circulation, accelerating healing and recovery.[90]

Another type of magnetic therapy is the PEMF (pulsed electromagnetic) mat. It works by sending short bursts of pulsed electromagnetic fields through your body, impacting the organs, bones, tissues and cells. These pulses stimulate healthy growth and activity in the cells, hopefully helping your body's natural healing processes occur. PEMF mats are considered by the manufacturers to be natural, safe, non-invasive ways to promote optimal health.

---

[89] *Root Causes*. (n.d.). Tennant Institute.
[90] Paul. (2017, May 16). *Does Magnetic Therapy Work?* Health and Care.

According to Biobalance, manufacturer of PEMF devices, the benefits can include "healing of bone and soft tissue, improving circulation, increasing immune function, positive impact on quality sleep, and offering relief from pain."[91] According to another PEMF manufacturer, Casaroma Wellness, "Increased calcium transport stimulates the repair and growth of cartilage, while at the same time decreasing pain." For this reason, Casaroma recommend the use of PEMF mats for sufferers of osteoporosis.[92]

These mats are very expensive and most likely used by wealthy people and professional athletes for recovery. It would be enlightening to find some up to date medical research in this area that one could trust. Given some very capable doctors tend to athletes at top sports clubs, whether it be American football, baseball, or football, these doctors wouldn't put their athletes at risk. However, that doesn't necessarily mean that the treatment has significant recovery potential.

Magnetism and body scanning

There is incredible scientific validation for magnetic scanning equipment. Magnetic resonance imaging (MRI) and fMRI scanners are incredibly important devices used today to identify issues that might be going on within our bodies. They are only two types of many different modern scanners that have completely revolutionised the way we can look at our bodies and understand how medicines or treatments work.

The MRI can scan parts of the body that can't be seen as well by X-rays, CT scans or ultrasounds. For example, MRI scans can help doctors to see inside joints, cartilage, ligaments, muscles and tendons, which makes it especially helpful for detecting various sports injuries.

---

[91] Dios, L. (2020, September 15). *How to Use PEMF Mats*. BioBalance PEMF.
[92] Casaroma Wellness. (2021, January 13). *The iMRS - Pulsed Magnetic Resonance Stimulation Mat*.

MRI is also used to examine internal body structures and diagnose a variety of disorders, such as strokes, tumours, aneurysms, spinal cord injuries, multiple sclerosis and eye or inner ear problems. It is also widely used in research to measure brain structure and function, among other things.

The way an MRI scan works is by applying a strong magnetic field that aligns with proton spins in our body's water molecules. The scanner produces a radio frequency current that creates a varying magnetic field. The protons absorb the energy from the magnetic field and flip their spins. When the field is turned off, the protons gradually return to their normal spin, a process called precession. The return process produces a radio signal that can be measured by receivers in the scanner and made into an image.[93]

fMRI scanning is the video version of an MRI scanner, but the resolution isn't quite as detailed. Still, fMRI is excellent for use in scanning our brain activity, as it may detect abnormalities within the brain that cannot be found with other imaging techniques.[94]

The level of understanding we now have about our bodies, simply from the successful introduction of MRI scanning into our healthcare systems, has allowed medical science to advance incredibly quickly. We can now see and understand the workings of our bodies in such extraordinary medical detail.

MRI scanners are being made to see at even greater detail or resolution. The most powerful machines can have magnets that weigh over 100 tonnes, with a resolution that can be as fine as 0.5 millimetres in some research MRI machines — enough to discern the functional units inside the human cortex and perhaps see for the first time how information flows between collections of neurons in a live human brain. Part of the scientific breakthrough has also been how to make this technology and scanner safe, especially given the powerful magnetic fields being used.

[93] Lewis, T. (2017, August 12). *What is an MRI (Magnetic Resonance Imaging)?* Livescience.Com.
[94] Acr, R. A. (2018, July 16). *Magnetic Resonance, Functional (fMRI) - Brain.* Radiologyinfo.Org.

This technology is finding more funding given how successful it is, and so we can expect at least twice the resolution from the next generation.

While MRI scanners are amazing in and of themselves, technology is continuing to advance at a rapid rate, and there are new scanners that take us to the edge of optical physics that could eventually replace the MRI scanner. A rather astounding inventor, Mary Lou Jepsen, gave a TED talk about her new technologies that use light, sound and advanced machine learning to see inside our bodies. This can enable us to track any potential tumour growths, and measure neural activity. Her new technology can see up to 1,000 times the scale of an MRI scanner. At this level of detail, we could replace the MRI machine with a cheaper, more efficient system. Mary Lou Jepsen's goal is to make these scanning devices a lot smaller and less expensive so that they can even be incorporated into a wearable device such as a helmet, belt, wristband, chest strap or sports bra. It is new technologies like these that demonstrate just how quickly we are developing in this field, with better tools to treat ourselves at home or on the go, without necessarily having to pay a visit to the hospital.

CHAPTER 12:
THE ROLE OF MEDITATION TO REGULATE OUR BODY

Meditation can be defined as a set of techniques that are intended to encourage a heightened state of awareness and focused attention. Meditation is also a consciousness-changing technique that has been shown to have a wide number of benefits on psychological well-being.[95]

Meditation is thought to be a key component in cultivating a calm and positive attitude and mental state. For many years, successful personalities such as Oprah Winfrey, Paul McCartney, Jerry Seinfeld and Tom Hanks have been open about their meditation practice and the benefits it brings them, and it is becoming increasingly widespread thanks to popular apps and programmes by companies like Headspace. Headspace recently released some study results, where they showed that 10 days of Headspace reduced stress by 14%, 3 weeks of Headspace increased compassion by 21%, and 10 days of Headspace reduced irritability by 27%. Not bad in my opinion, and probably worth the 10 minutes a day.[96]

What is meditation after all?

Meditation can be performed in many different ways and there are various techniques and practices that may work better for you than others. There are hundreds of free guided meditations online or in free podcasts or with phone apps. I've used Headspace for a long-time now, and so wanted to summarise its beginner program. The process is typically as follows:

[95] Cherry, K. (2020, September 1). *How Meditation Impacts Your Mind and Body*. Verywell Mind.
[96] *Researching Meditation and Mindfulness*. (2021). Headspace.

- Sit in a comfortable position in a space that is of a steady temperature. Try to find a spot that is away from loud noises and the possibility of interruptions, if only for ten to twenty minutes.
- Close your eyes, and focus on breathing steadily through your nose, into your stomach and out again through the nose.
- Allow your breath to return to its natural steady pace and continue to focus your attention on it.
- The idea is to calm your mind and tune out any pressing thoughts or responsibilities, giving your mind a well-needed rest. However, your mind is likely to wander – a lot. This is completely normal, and it takes time to train the mind to relax and quieten. Simply notice where your thoughts are going, then let those thoughts go and return your focus to your breath. It doesn't matter if you need to do this a hundred times in one ten minute sitting. Meditation is a practice, and it may take a few (or a lot of) attempts before your mind eventually slows.

Early meditation sessions can be as short as five minutes long, but as your mind begins to adapt, you may want to make your sessions a little longer. Many people meditate for up to an hour a day, but just ten or twenty minutes may be enough for you. The key is to listen to your intuition for what works best for you.

What are the effects of meditation?

It has been found that, during the process of meditation, accumulated stresses are removed, energy is increased, and health is positively affected overall. Research has confirmed a myriad of health benefits associated with the practice of meditation, so that after your sessions there are positive signs of stress reduction, decreased anxiety, decreased depression, reduction in pain, improved memory, and increased efficiency. Not only that, but physiological benefits include reduced blood pressure and heart rate, decreased metabolism, and increased blood flow to the brain.

The reason is cited to be that meditation increases blood flow in the frontal and anterior regions of the brain, increasing the efficiency of the brain's performance.

Meditation and the brain

A study by UCLA found that people who had meditated long-term had better-preserved brains than people who hadn't meditated. Participants in the study who had been meditating for an average of 20 years had more grey matter volume throughout the brain. And although older meditators still had some volume loss compared to younger meditators, it wasn't as pronounced as the non-meditators. According to study author, Florian Kurth, "We expected rather small and distinct effects located in some of the regions that had previously been associated with meditating. Instead, what we actually observed was a widespread effect of meditation that encompassed regions throughout the entire brain."[97] Increasing grey matter in the brain is important for slowing cognitive degeneration that can lead to neurodegenerative diseases such as Alzheimer's and dementia.[98]

Another study carried out by Yale University found that mindfulness meditation decreases activity in the default mode network (DMN), the brain network responsible for mind-wandering and self-referential. Self-referential rumination or mind-wandering is thought to be associated with lower levels of happiness, and a tendency to worry about the past and future. Several studies have shown that meditation, through its quieting effect on the DMN, appears to reduce this mind-wandering activity day-to-day.[99]

Not only is meditation thought to be useful in preserving brain quality and functionality, but it is also suggested it can lead to fundamental changes in the brain, positively affecting our ability to learn, remember and regulate emotion. It is also thought that meditation could reduce levels of anxiety as well as rival medicinal treatments targeting depression and anxiety and help with addiction.[100]

---

[97] Sharma, H. (2015, September). *Meditation: Process and effects*. PubMed Central (PMC).
[98] Wheeler, M. (2015, February 5). *Forever young: Meditation might slow the age-related loss of gray matter in the brain, say UCLA researchers*. UCLA.
[99] Garrison, K. A., Zeffiro, T. A., Scheinost, D., Constable, R. T., & Brewer, J. A. (2015). *Meditation leads to reduced default mode network activity beyond an active task.* Cognitive, Affective, & Behavioral Neuroscience
[100] Walton, A. G. (2021, April 10). *7 Ways Meditation Can Actually Change The Brain*. Forbes.

Meditation and ageing

As we've discussed earlier in the book, inflammation is a key factor in the ageing of our bodies. Meditation has been found to protect people from the inflammatory stress response.[101] Not only that but it has also been shown that meditators seem to benefit from increased telomerase activity to support healthy telomeres, which we know is another important factor in bodily function and long-term health.[102]

As yet, there has been no evidence to suggest that meditation is bad for us. Studies into the benefits of meditation have so far only been positive. So in my view, there is nothing to lose from giving it a try, and potentially, a huge amount to gain.

[101] *Beneficial Effects of Meditation on Inflammation*. (2020, October 5). The Institute for Functional Medicine.
[102] Smith, J. A. (2021, March 9). *10 Things We Know About the Science of Meditation*. Mindful.

CHAPTER 13:

WE WILL ALL GET LONG LIFE EXPECTANCIES

We've explored many different areas that relate to our present and future health, ranging from diagnostic developments to cell manipulation and nurturing treatments, all of which could have a certain and positive impact on our lifespan. The major effects that we will likely experience though is an increased healthspan, the number of healthy and active years we generate for ourselves. I hope that all this is leading you towards a mindset that is more open to the idea of living longer than you perhaps expected to.

While there are plenty of age-slowing and rejuvenation options currently available to the wealthy, most people who are able to receive modern healthcare will likely benefit too.

There is a strong likelihood that we will live longer than our parents and grandparents, simply because of medical advancement, hopefully supported by a better understanding of lifestyle and health practices.

The average lifespan increases by six years with every new generation. So, for example, 80 years of age on average, becomes 86 years on average for the next generation, and then 92 for the generation after that. The lifespan of humans will continue to improve well into the hundreds, and the healthspan, those glorious years of being mostly disease-free, are likely to extend throughout most of that lifespan.

Picking a new number to think of as a normal life expectancy is becoming harder, mostly because 100 may be too short, considering some of the findings explored in this book. Would it be unreasonable to suggest life expectancy for you, me, our children, our grandchildren, could be 120, 150 or more?

Living for another 20 years is going to be crucial to see some of the most astounding health discoveries come to light. There is every chance that we will be able to safely rejuvenate ourselves so that we can come to expect a 150-year lifespan as normal.

A 150-year lifespan would not only be long given our current viewpoint but also very long in terms of the advances that a person would live through. The pace of change and the new discoveries are increasing. I dream of what may come in another hundred years, and it gives me cause to want to shape the future for the better. That is the topic for another book. A topic that we should also start to consider as more relevant given we are likely to live into the long future.

Living to those (currently thought of as extreme) ages is not guaranteed, if only it was as simple as that. Living in good health to those ages won't happen if you don't take care of your health now. While scientific and medical developments are advancing rapidly and providing more and more ways in which we can treat and even eradicate serious health conditions, healthcare still may not be enough if we don't maintain a healthy baseline founded in exercise and good nutrition as well as complementary mental health practices. And if we look back to the Blue Zone communities, we would also do well to consider other factors such as social connectivity in preparing us for longer life.

As David Setboun, president of the Academy for Health and Lifespan Research said, "The main objective is to live *healthier* longer, and the side effect of that is you tend to live longer as well."[103]

If you are indeed prepared to change some of your lifestyle habits and health regimes, and you are dedicated to knowing and

---

[103] Stinson, L. (2020, August 18). *Our Average Life Expectancy Could Increase to 115 Years Very Soon*. Allure.

understanding the health status of your body, then you can expect to live a longer life than perhaps you'd expected. You might want to be open to some of the treatments and approaches that we've outlined, which is fantastic, and I implore you to do your own research and consult with your physician or your doctor.

Also, now is a good time to start thinking about those goals you didn't think you'd have time to achieve, the places you didn't think you'd be able to explore, the subjects you didn't think you'd have the brain health to study. It's time to reset your dreams and relax. You have time.

CONCLUSION

I started by recognising that there is such a large amount of information out in the world about health and longevity, and yet our current mindset is preventing us from outliving the current statistics. The problem is that there is a lot of different data available, and I've covered a wide range of pieces of the puzzle. Some of this will become clearer as medical practitioners summarise the most effective methods of healthcare. In the meantime, we need to make our own way with the information, and I think you're in a far better position now having understood the latest updates described in this book.

The other problem is that we still think we may only live to 70-something years, when in fact we could be expecting a far longer lifespan. Not only that, but we can also be much healthier for longer. We can see our bodies stay young for far longer than previously imaginable.

We've covered many ideas that have shown mindset is very important to adjust. A healthy mind and mindset will ensure you become healthier as an individual.

We've explored the importance of having a purpose and an understanding of our reason for living, as well as goals to help us achieve our dreams. And we also discussed how important it is to engage with the process as much as the goal itself.

We looked at the phenomenal discovery and identification of the Blue Zone communities and the common traits they share, which are all thought to contribute towards the longer lifespan of the inhabitants. It has been interesting that the long-life factors go beyond the common understanding of diet and exercise, to slowing down, employing moderation and nurturing a sense of community and closeness with family, friends and neighbours.

We took a glance at what the billionaire's choices are when it comes to expensive healthcare. These treatments and products won't remain out of our grasp forever, and these are clues as to what else could come down the line in terms of tools to help us better manage our health, and therefore our longevity. Many are affordable to those now that have modest wealth.

We discussed what ageing is, how the role of telomeres and senescent cells act in the ageing process, and we looked at new scientific breakthroughs that point to technological and medicinal advancements that we can all look forward to in the future. We also have discovered that our DNA can repair itself so long as we support those biological functions.

Supplements and energy-based treatments are two more interesting factors in health management and optimisation that we looked at.

There are supplements available now that are specifically taken to lower our biological age. NMN, Resveratrol, and Metformin work in ways to enhance our DNA repair mechanisms and could be recommended one day if safely studied and approved. Fasting or intermittent fasting have similar effects to these supplements – so long as you do this healthily. This is very easy to get wrong, so please consult with your doctor or physician before attempting any diet changes.

Mental health, we discovered, plays a crucial role in enhancing our overall wellness and likelihood of living longer. We discussed the value of therapy as well as meditation in supporting the health and stability of our minds.

One of the most exciting aspects of our understanding of ageing is that the latest science and future developments will completely reinvent our health treatments. We are going to have bespoke medicine, gene therapy, stem cell therapy and many more scientific advantages that will slow our ageing for decades. These breakthroughs may even lead to reversing our biological ageing to our prime health.

Whether you prefer the advantages of science and scanning, or meditation to improve your life, in my opinion, a combination of all of these will make the biggest difference.

And putting it all together will give you time. More time than you realised you had, more time to be healthy, more time to be with the people you love, as well as their future generations.

If you want to do one little thing that means you'll stay connected to this positive lifestyle, then join the community at www.howardeweller.com. We want to spread the message of longevity, and to provide quality information that is relevant to you.

And lastly, if you've liked this book and the messages about improving your life then please leave a review for other people to benefit too. Your feedback will help to spread the message of what's really possible for us, our friends and our families.

Thank you.

REFERENCES AND FURTHER READING

Introduction

1. Basaraba, S. (2020, April 24). How Has Longevity Changed Throughout History? Verywell Health. https://www.verywellhealth.com/longevity-throughout-history-2224054

2. Kamal, R. (2019, December 23). Health System Tracker. Health System Tracker. https://www.healthsystemtracker.org/chart-collection/u-s-life-expectancy-compare-countries/#item-le_life-expectancy-at-birth-in-years-2017_dec-2019-update

3. Raypole, C. (2020, August 31). Time Anxiety. Healthline. https://www.healthline.com/health/mental-health/time-anxiety

4. Kluger, J. (2015, February 12). How Your Mindset Can Change How You Age. Time. https://time.com/3706720/how-your-mindset-can-change-how-you-age/

Chapter 1

5. Dweck, C. (2017b). Mindset - Updated Edition: Changing The Way You think To Fulfil Your Potential (6th ed.). Little, Brown Book Group.

6. Dweck, C. (2016, January 13). What Having a "Growth Mindset" Actually Means. Harvard Business Review. https://hbr.org/2016/01/what-having-a-growth-mindset-actually-means

7. Gottfredson, R., & Reina, C. (2020, January 17). To Be a Great Leader, You Need the Right Mindset. Harvard Business Review. https://hbr.org/2020/01/to-be-a-great-leader-you-need-the-right-mindset

8. Lee, L. O. (2019, September 10). Optimism is associated with exceptional longevity in 2 epidemiologic cohorts of men and women. PubMed. https://pubmed.ncbi.nlm.nih.gov/31451635

9. James, P. (2018, July 3). Optimism and Healthy Ageing in Women. PubMed. https://pubmed.ncbi.nlm.nih.gov/30573140/

Chapter 2

10. Erin, S. (2019, September 20). Your "Why" Matters: The 10 Benefits of Knowing Your Purpose in Life. Goalcast. https://www.goalcast.com/2017/05/17/10-benefits-of-knowing-your-purpose-in-life/

11. Sillers, J. (2017, July 19). Why more ambitious goals are more likely to help. The Orange Dot. https://www.headspace.com/blog/2017/05/15/ambitious-goals/

12. Infoplease. (2020, August 5). Life Expectancy by Age, 1850-2011. https://www.infoplease.com/us/health-statistics/life-expectancy-age-1850-2011

13. Frost, N. (2018, September 4). Two Presidents Died on the Same July 4: Coincidence or Something More? HISTORY. https://www.history.com/news/july-4-two-presidents-died-same-day-coincidence

14. Clear, J. (2020, February 4). Forget About Setting Goals. Focus on This Instead. James Clear. https://jamesclear.com/goals-systems

15. Zupanic, M. (2019, September 20). How To Find Your Passion. Goalcast. https://www.goalcast.com/2016/09/13/how-to-find-your-passion/

16. Hari, J. (2019). Lost Connections: Why You're Depressed and How to Find Hope (Reprint ed.). Bloomsbury Publishing.

Chapter 3

17. Blue Zones—Live Longer, Better. (2021, May 6). Blue Zones. https://www.bluezones.com/

18. Koroshetz, K. (2019, December 18). The Geographic Areas Where People Live the Longest—and Clues as to Why. Goop. https://goop.com/wellness/health/the-geographic-areas-where-people-live-the-longest-and-clues-as-to-why/

19. Koroshetz, K. (2019, December 18). The Geographic Areas Where People Live the Longest—and Clues as to Why. Goop. https://goop.com/wellness/health/the-geographic-areas-where-people-live-the-longest-and-clues-as-to-why/

20. Kotifani, A. (2020, June 2). Fasting for Health and Longevity: Nobel Prize-Winning Research on Cell Ageing. Blue Zones. https://www.bluezones.com/2018/10/fasting-for-health-and-longevity-nobel-prize-winning-research-on-cell-ageing/

21. Walker, M. (2018). Why We Sleep: Unlocking the Power of Sleep and Dreams. Scribner.

22. Four Pillar Freedom. (2019, November 13). Why We Sleep by Matthew Walker: Summary and Notes. https://fourpillarfreedom.com/why-we-sleep-by-matthew-walker/

23. Four Pillar Freedom. (2019, November 13). Why We Sleep by Matthew Walker: Summary and Notes. https://fourpillarfreedom.com/why-we-sleep-by-matthew-walker/

24. Suni, E. (2020, October 23). How Sleep Works. Sleep Foundation. https://www.sleepfoundation.org/how-sleep-works

25. Gilbert, S. (2019, November 18). The Importance of Community and Mental Health | NAMI: National Alliance on Mental Illness. NAMI: National Alliance on Mental Illness. https://nami.org/Blogs/NAMI-Blog/November-2019/The-Importance-of-Community-and-Mental-Health

Chapter 4

26. Diamandis, P. H. (2020, October 18). Increase your healthspan, now. Diamandis. https://www.diamandis.com/blog/increase-healthspan-now

27. Diamandis, P. H. (2020, October 18). Increase your healthspan, now. Diamandis. https://www.diamandis.com/blog/increase-healthspan-now

28. Harvard Health. (2020, June 17). Understanding your health status. https://www.health.harvard.edu/staying-healthy/living-wills-7

29. Hildreth, C. (2020, October 12). Can We Extend the Human Lifespan With Regenerative Medicine? BioInformant. https://bioinformant.com/regenerative-medicine/

30. Finance, A. (2020, May 22). How Billionaires Plan to Live Forever | ABC Finance Ltd. ABC Finance. https://abcfinance.co.uk/blog/how-billionaires-plan-to-live-forever/

31. Shen, J. (2019, May 30). Effects of light on ageing and longevity. PubMed. https://www.ncbi.nlm.nih.gov/pmc/articles/PMC6663583/

32. Johnstone, D. (2016, January 11). Turning On Lights to Stop Neurodegeneration: The Potential of Near Infrared Light Therapy in Alzheimer's and Parkinson's Disease. PubMed Central (PMC). https://www.ncbi.nlm.nih.gov/pmc/articles/PMC4707222/

33. Casaroma Wellness. (2021, January 13). The iMRS - Pulsed Magnetic Resonance Stimulation Mat. https://casaromawellness.com/wp/imrs-pulsed-magnetic-resonance-stimulation-mat/

34. Finance, A. (2020, May 22). How Billionaires Plan to Live Forever | ABC Finance Ltd. ABC Finance. https://abcfinance.co.uk/blog/how-billionaires-plan-to-live-forever/

35. Finance, A. (2020, May 22). How Billionaires Plan to Live Forever | ABC Finance Ltd. ABC Finance. https://abcfinance.co.uk/blog/how-billionaires-plan-to-live-forever/

Chapter 5

36. Adam, D. (2021, April 30). What if ageing weren't inevitable, but a curable disease? MIT Technology Review. https://www.technologyreview.com/2019/08/19/133357/what-if-ageing-werent-inevitable-but-a-curable-disease

37. Marsh, A. (2021, May 24). *Olympian, actor. . . wealth manager? Meet Michel de Carvalho, one half of Britain's ninth richest couple.* Spear's Magazine. https://www.spearswms.com/michel-de-carvalho-spears/

38. Australian Academy of Science, & Graves, J. (2018, October 10). What are telomeres? Australian Academy of Science.

https://www.science.org.au/curious/people-medicine/what-are-telomeres

39.   Shay, J. W. (2000, October 1). Hayflick, his limit, and cellular ageing. Nature Reviews Molecular Cell Biology. https://www.nature.com/articles/35036093

40.   Scharping, N. (2020, August 11). Senolytics: A New Weapon in the War on Ageing. Discover Magazine. https://www.discovermagazine.com/health/senolytics-a-new-weapon-in-the-war-on-ageing

41.   Scharping, N. (2020, August 11). Senolytics: A New Weapon in the War on Ageing. Discover Magazine. https://www.discovermagazine.com/health/senolytics-a-new-weapon-in-the-war-on-ageing

42.   Whittemore, K. (2019, July 23). Telomere shortening rate predicts species life span. PNAS. https://www.pnas.org/content/116/30/15122

Chapter 6

43.   Ross, B. (2021, March 7). Trends Transforming The Precision Medicine Industry In 2021 from. Linchpin SEO. https://linchpinseo.com/trends-in-precision-medicine/

44.   Reader, R. (2019, December 16). Amazon and Apple will be our doctors in the future, says tech guru Peter Diamandis. Fast Company. https://www.fastcompany.com/90440921/amazon-and-apple-will-be-our-doctors-in-the-future-says-tech-guru-peter-diamandis

45.   What are genome editing and CRISPR-Cas9?: MedlinePlus Genetics. (n.d.). MedlinePlus. Retrieved May 11, 2021, from https://medlineplus.gov/genetics/understanding/genomicresearch/genomeediting/

46.   What is CRISPR? (n.d.). New Scientist. Retrieved May 11, 2021, from https://www.newscientist.com/definition/what-is-crispr/

47.   Butera, S. (2018, April 23). CAR-T: trailblazing the path from clinical development to the clinic. Gene Therapy. https://www.nature.com/articles/s41434-018-0013-z

48.   Diamandis, P. H. (n.d.). 100 years old will be the new 60. Diamandis. Retrieved May 11, 2021, from https://www.diamandis.com/blog/100-new-60

49.   Hale, C. (2020, September 21). Illumina to pay $8B to reacquire cancer blood test maker Grail, with all eyes on 2021. FierceBiotech. https://www.fiercebiotech.com/medtech/illumina-to-pay-8b-to-reacquire-cancer-blood-test-maker-grail-all-eyes-2021

50.   Pennisi, E. (2021, March 18). 'Total game changer': Pinpointing gene activity in tissues is aiding. Science | AAAS. https://www.sciencemag.org/news/2021/03/total-game-changer-pinpointing-gene-activity-tissues-aiding-studies-covid-19-alzheimer

51.   Cross, R. (2018, July 30). Meet the exosome, the rising star in drug delivery. Chemical & Engineering News. https://cen.acs.org/business/start-ups/Meet-exosome-rising-star-drug/96/i31

52.   How the vaccine works. (n.d.). Imperial College London. Retrieved May 11, 2021, from https://www.imperial.ac.uk/covid-19-vaccine-trial/vaccine-science/

Chapter 7

53.   Sinclair, D., & LaPlante, M. D. (2019). *Lifespan: Why We Age—and Why We Don't* Have To (Illustrated ed.). Atria Books.

54.   Blackburn, E., & Epel, E. (2018). The Telomere Effect: A Revolutionary Approach to Living Younger, Healthier, Longer (Illustrated ed.). Grand Central Publishing.

55.   Epel, E. (2017, February 13). How to Create the Ideal Diet for Telomere Heath. ELLE. https://www.elle.com/life-love/a42611/telomere-treats-oh-what-to-eat/

56.   Ware, M. R. (2018, May 29). How can antioxidants benefit our health? Medical News Today. https://www.medicalnewstoday.com/articles/301506

57.   Eske, J. (2019, August 30). 4 natural ways to increase glutathione. Medical News Today. https://www.medicalnewstoday.com/articles/326196#possible-benefits

58.   Tucker, L. A. (2018, April 1). Dietary Fiber and Telomere Length in 5674 U.S. Adults: An NHANES Study of Biological Ageing. PubMed Central (PMC). https://www.ncbi.nlm.nih.gov/pmc/articles/PMC5946185/

59.   Watson, K. (2020, March 26). Benefits of Inulin. Healthline. https://www.healthline.com/health/food-nutrition/top-inulin-benefits#benefits-of-inulin

60.   Tucker, L. A. (2018b, April 1). Dietary Fiber and Telomere Length in 5674 U.S. Adults: An NHANES Study of Biological Ageing. PubMed Central (PMC). https://www.ncbi.nlm.nih.gov/pmc/articles/PMC5946185/#B45-nutrients-10-00400

61.   Blagosklonny, M. V. (2019). Fasting and rapamycin: diabetes versus benevolent glucose intolerance. Cell Death & Disease, 10(8). https://doi.org/10.1038/s41419-019-1822-8

62.   Nall, R. M. (2019, September 19). What to know about nitric oxide supplements. Medical News Today. https://www.medicalnewstoday.com/articles/326381#how-they-work

63.   Moore, R. (2021, January 2). Is It Possible to Lengthen Telomeres With Diet & Exercise? Visual Impact Fitness. https://visualimpactfitness.com/lengthen-telomeres-diet-exercise/

64.   What Diet is Best for Me? Paleo? Keto? Vegan? (2018, June 29). Viome. https://www.viome.com/blog/paleo-keto-vegan-what-perfect-diet-you

Chapter 8

65. What is NMN? (2021, May 11). NMN.com.
https://www.nmn.com/precursors/what-is-nmn

66. Everything You Always Wanted to Know About Metformin, But Were Afraid to Ask. (2021, March 18). DiaTribe.
https://diatribe.org/everything-you-always-wanted-know-about-metformin-were-afraid-ask

67. Metformin in Longevity Study (MILES). - Full Text View - ClinicalTrials.gov. (n.d.). Clinical Trials. Retrieved May 11, 2021, from https://clinicaltrials.gov/ct2/show/NCT02432287

68. Palliyaguru, D. L., Minor, R. K., Mitchell, S. J., Palacios, H. H., Licata, J. J., Ward, T. M., Abulwerdi, G., Elliott, P., Westphal, C., Ellis, J. L., Sinclair, D. A., Price, N. L., Bernier, M., & de Cabo, R. (2020). Combining a High Dose of Metformin With the SIRT1 Activator, SRT1720, Reduces Life Span in Aged Mice Fed a High-Fat Diet. The Journals of Gerontology: Series A, 75(11), 2037–2041.
https://doi.org/10.1093/gerona/glaa148

69. Blagosklonny, M. V. (2019). Fasting and rapamycin: diabetes versus benevolent glucose intolerance. Nature.
https://www.nature.com/articles/s41419-019-1822-8.pdf

70. Harvard Health. (2012, February 3). Resveratrol—the hype continues.
https://www.health.harvard.edu/blog/resveratrol-the-hype-continues-201202034189

71. McDermott, A. (2018, September 18). What Is Phosphatidylcholine and How Is It Used? Healthline.
https://www.healthline.com/health/food-nutrition/phosphatidylcholine

72. Garma, J. (2019, July 19). 7 Phosphatidylcholine Benefits That Can Improve Your Long-term Health. ProHealth Longevity.
https://www.prohealthlongevity.com/blogs/control-how-you-age/7-phosphatidylcholine-benefits-that-can-improve-your-long-term-health

73. Phosphatidylcholine: Health Benefits, Uses, Side Effects, Dosage & Interactions. (2019, September 17). RxList.
https://www.rxlist.com/phosphatidylcholine/supplements.htm

Chapter 9

74. Wikipedia contributors. (2021, May 6). Stem-cell therapy. Wikipedia.
https://en.wikipedia.org/wiki/Stem-cell_therapy

75. NHS website. (2020, May 5). Stem cell and bone marrow transplants. Nhs.Uk. https://www.nhs.uk/conditions/stem-cell-transplant/

76. Stem cell (cell replacement) therapy. (n.d.). European Parkinson's Disease Association. Retrieved May 11, 2021, from https://www.epda.eu.com/living-well/therapies/surgical-treatments/stem-cell-cell-replacement-therapy/

77. Parkinson's disease: how could stem cells help? (n.d.). Eurostemcell. Retrieved May 11, 2021, from

https://www.eurostemcell.org/parkinsons-disease-how-could-stem-cells-help

78.   Stem cell (cell replacement) therapy. (n.d.). European Parkinson's Disease Association. Retrieved May 11, 2021, from https://www.epda.eu.com/living-well/therapies/surgical-treatments/stem-cell-cell-replacement-therapy/

79.   Evangelou, C. (2020, January 17). Using stem cells to reverse ageing? Longevity.Technology. https://www.longevity.technology/using-stem-cells-to-reverse-ageing/

Chapter 10

80.   Shields, G. S. (2020, October 1). Psychosocial Interventions and Immune System Function: A Systematic Review and Meta-analysis of Randomized Clinical Trials. PubMed. https://pubmed.ncbi.nlm.nih.gov/32492090/

81.   Hollstadt, N. (2020, November 22). David Hoy and Associates. David Hoy & Associates. https://davidhoy.com/5-long-term-benefits-of-therapy/

82.   NHS website. (2021, February 25). Overview - Cognitive behavioural therapy (CBT). Nhs.Uk. https://www.nhs.uk/mental-health/talking-therapies-medicine-treatments/talking-therapies-and-counselling/cognitive-behavioural-therapy-cbt/overview/

83.   Good Therapy Editor Team. (n.d.). Psychodynamic Therapy. Good Therapy. Retrieved May 11, 2021, from https://www.goodtherapy.org/learn-about-therapy/types/psychodynamic

84.   What Is Postpartum PTSD? (2020, May 27). Goop. https://goop.com/wellness/parenthood/postpartum-ptsd/

85.   Harvard Health. (2019, October 16). If you are happy and you know it... you may live longer. https://www.health.harvard.edu/blog/if-you-are-happy-and-you-know-it-you-may-live-longer-2019101618020

86.   Lee, L. O. (2019, September 10). Optimism is associated with exceptional longevity in 2 epidemiologic cohorts of men and women. PubMed. https://pubmed.ncbi.nlm.nih.gov/31451635/

87.   Harvard Health. (2019b, October 16). If you are happy and you know it. . . you may live longer. https://www.health.harvard.edu/blog/if-you-are-happy-and-you-know-it-you-may-live-longer-2019101618020

Chapter 11

88.   Bach, M. (n.d.). What Are Energy Therapies? Taking Charge of Your Health & Wellbeing. Retrieved May 11, 2021, from https://www.takingcharge.csh.umn.edu/what-are-energy-therapies

89.   Root Causes. (n.d.). Tennant Institute. Retrieved May 11, 2021, from https://tennantinstitute.com/root-causes/

90.   Paul. (2017, May 16). Does Magnetic Therapy Work? Health and Care. https://www.healthandcare.co.uk/blog/does-magnetic-therapy-work.html

91.   Dios, L. (2020, September 15). How to Use PEMF Mats. BioBalance PEMF. https://biobalancepemf.com/how-to-use-pemf-mats/

92.   Casaroma Wellness. (2021, January 13). The iMRS - Pulsed Magnetic Resonance Stimulation Mat. https://casaromawellness.com/wp/imrs-pulsed-magnetic-resonance-stimulation-mat/

93.   Lewis, T. (2017, August 12). What is an MRI (Magnetic Resonance Imaging)? Livescience.Com. https://www.livescience.com/39074-what-is-an-mri.html

94.   Acr, R. A. (2018, July 16). Magnetic Resonance, Functional (fMRI) - Brain. Radiologyinfo.Org. https://www.radiologyinfo.org/en/info/fmribrain

Chapter 12

95.   Cherry, K. (2020, September 1). How Meditation Impacts Your Mind and Body. Verywell Mind. https://www.verywellmind.com/what-is-meditation-2795927

96.   Researching Meditation and Mindfulness. (2021). Headspace. https://www.headspace.com/science/meditation-research

97.   Sharma, H. (2015, September). Meditation: Process and effects. PubMed Central (PMC). https://www.ncbi.nlm.nih.gov/pmc/articles/PMC4895748/

98.   Wheeler, M. (2015, February 5). Forever young: Meditation might slow the age-related loss of gray matter in the brain, say UCLA researchers. UCLA. https://newsroom.ucla.edu/releases/forever-young-meditation-might-slow-the-age-related-loss-of-gray-matter-in-the-brain-say-ucla-researchers

99.   Garrison, K. A., Zeffiro, T. A., Scheinost, D., Constable, R. T., & Brewer, J. A. (2015). Meditation leads to reduced default mode network activity beyond an active task. Cognitive, Affective, & Behavioral Neuroscience, 15(3), 712–720. https://doi.org/10.3758/s13415-015-0358-3

100.   Walton, A. G. (2021, April 10). 7 Ways Meditation Can Actually Change The Brain. Forbes. https://www.forbes.com/sites/alicegwalton/2015/02/09/7-ways-meditation-can-actually-change-the-brain/?sh=dc3cce714658

101.   Beneficial Effects of Meditation on Inflammation. (2020, October 5). The Institute for Functional Medicine. https://www.ifm.org/news-insights/lifestyle-effects-meditation-inflammation/

102.   Smith, J. A. (2021, March 9). 10 Things We Know About the Science of Meditation. Mindful. https://www.mindful.org/10-things-we-know-about-the-science-of-meditation/

Chapter 13

103.   Stinson, L. (2020, August 18). *Our Average Life Expectancy Could Increase to 115 Years Very Soon*. Allure. https://www.allure.com/story/the-future-of-ageing

ADDITIONAL REFERENCES:

Introduction
104.   Butler, R. N. (2008). The Longevity Revolution: The Benefits and Challenges of Living a Long Life (1st ed.). PublicAffairs.

Chapter 1

105.   Sanderson, C. A. (2019). The Positive Shift: Mastering Mindset to Improve Happiness, Health, and Longevity. BenBella Books.

Chapter 4

106.   Corbyn, Z. (2018, February 15). Live for ever: Scientists say they'll soon extend life 'well beyond 120.' The Guardian. https://www.theguardian.com/science/2015/jan/11/-sp-live-forever-extend-life-calico-google-longevity
107.   Shead, S. (2019, August 21). Billionaire Backs U.K. Startup Trying To Extend Human Life Spans. Forbes. https://www.forbes.com/sites/samshead/2019/08/19/billionaire-backs-uk-startup-trying-to-extend-human-lifespans/?sh=7f8145ff5f03
108.   Friend, T. (2019, July 9). Silicon Valley's Quest to Live Forever. The New Yorker. https://www.newyorker.com/magazine/2017/04/03/silicon-valleys-quest-to-live-forever
109.   Barclay, T. (2021b, April 11). Finding the Best DNA Health Test. Innerbody. https://www.innerbody.com/dna-testing/dna-health-testing
110.   Learn How to Determine Your Cellular Age. (2021). Teloyears. https://teloyears.com/how-teloyears-works.html

Chapter 12

111. Tennant, J. L. (2010). Healing is Voltage: The Handbook, 3rd Edition (3rd ed.). CreateSpace Independent Publishing Platform.

112. Efron, Z., Olien, D., Barrett, J., Gmelich, G., Henson, C., Simpkin, M., Volk-Weiss, B. (Executive Producers). (2020). Down to Earth [TV Series]. The Nacelle Company.

Chapter 13

113. *Lifespan is continuing to increase regardless of socioeconomic factors, Stanford researchers find.* (2018, November 6). Stanford University. https://news.stanford.edu/press-releases/2018/11/06/lifespan-increasing-people-live-65/

Printed in Great Britain
by Amazon